Standard Comprehensive
Training for Estheticians Exam Review

chp. 33   100%
chp. 34   98%
chp. 21   98%
chp. 22   100%
chp. 23   100%
chp. 24   100%
chp 25

Switched
weeks
April 21st — chp. 35 & 36   Nicole from Rocco
April 28th — chp. 27 & 28   whole food facials

Chp. 35
Chp. 36
Chp. 27
Chp. 28

Standard Comprehensive
Training for Estheticians Exam Review

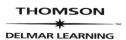

THOMSON

———*———™

DELMAR LEARNING

Australia   Canada   Mexico   Singapore   Spain   United Kingdom   United States

NOTICE TO THE READER

Publisher does not warrant or guarantee any of the products described herein or perform any independent analysis in connection with any of the product information contained herein. Publisher does not assume, and expressly disclaims, any obligation to obtain and include information other than that provided to it by the manufacturer.

The reader is expressly warned to consider and adopt all safety precautions that might be indicated by the activities herein and to avoid all potential hazards. By following the instructions contained herein, the reader willingly assumes all risks in connection with such instructions.

The Publisher makes no representation or warranties of any kind, including but not limited to, the warranties of fitness for particular purpose or merchantability, nor are any such representations implied with respect to the material set forth herein, and the publisher takes no responsibility with respect to such material. The Publisher shall not be liable for any special, consequential, or exemplary damages resulting, in whole or in part, from the readers' use of, or reliance upon, this material.

Table of Contents

Part VI - Advanced Sciences

Part VII - Advanced Skin Care

Part VIII - Epilation

Part IX - Makeup Artistry

Part X - The Spa Body Treatments

Part XI - Advanced Clinical Skin Care

Foreword

Milady's Standard Comprehensive Training for Estheticians Exam Review has been revised to follow very closely the type of skin care questions most frequently used by states and by the national testing, conducted under the auspices of the National-Interstate Council of State Boards of Cosmetology.

This review book is designed to be of major assistance to students in preparing for the state license examinations. In addition, its regular use in the classroom will serve as an important aid in the understanding of all subjects taught in cosmetology schools and required in the practice of cosmetology.

The exclusive concentration on multiple-choice test items reflects the fact that all state board examinations and national testing examinations are confined to this type of question.

Questions on the state board examinations in different states will not be exactly like these and may not touch upon all the information covered in this review. But students who diligently study and practice their work as taught in the classroom and who use this book for test preparation and review should receive higher grades on both classroom and license examinations.

Chapter *1*

A JOURNEY THROUGH TIME: ESTHETICS THEN AND NOW

1. Esthetics finds its roots in:
   a) French
   b) Greek
   c) Egyptian
   d) none of the above are correct   _____

2. In ancient times, beeswax was commonly used as it is today for:
   a) cooking
   b) bathing
   c) making candles
   d) dyeing fabric   _____

3. The theory that microorganisms were the cause of disease and infection came from:
   a) alchemists
   b) Louis Pasteur
   c) Hippocrates
   d) Galenus   _____

4. Ocean water therapies are known as:
   a) fangotherapy
   b) thalasotherapy
   c) hydrotherapy
   d) none of the above are correct   _____

5. The circadian rhythm, discovered by the Chinese, can be described as:
   a) vital life force flowing through the body
   b) the body's natural 24-hour cycle
   c) a person's constitution, temperament, and health
   d) the science of life   _____

6. Some of earliest cosmetic, fragrance, and herbal preparations were invented by the:
   a) Egyptians
   b) Greeks
   c) Romans
   d) Indians   _____

7. Vermilion was used for:
   a) eyeliner
   b) perfume
   c) coloring wigs and hair
   d) lip and cheek color   _____

8. The ancient practice of Ayurveda, revived in modern spas today, is based on:
   a) the flow of vital energy through the body
   b) applying shea butter for healing
   c) the healing properties of mineral springs and vapor caves
   d) treating the whole person to heal the mind, body, and spirit   _____

9. During the Victorian era, which was NOT true?
   a) makeup and elaborate clothing were discouraged
   b) both men and women were plain and austere
   c) beauty masks and packs made of fresh ingredients were used
   d) all of the above are true   _____

10. Western medicine is known as:
    a) homeopathy
    b) allopathic
    c) technical chemistry
    d) none of the above are correct   _____

11. The development of witch hazel was used in the 19th century for:
    a) gunshot wounds
    b) sunburn
    c) lesions
    d) all of the above are correct   _____

12. The first waterproof mascara was launched by:
    a) Aida Grey
    b) Elizabeth Arden
    c) Helena Rubinstein
    d) Max Factor   _____

13. The study of the physiological and therapeutic properties of mineral waters upon the body is known as:
    a) hydrolysis
    b) hydriatics
    c) hydrotherapy
    d) hydroponics   _____

Chapter 2

ANATOMY AND PHYSIOLOGY OF THE SKIN

1. The branch of anatomical science that deals with the overall health and well-being of the skin is called:
   a) dermatology
   b) cosmetics
   c) esthetics
   d) cytology

   C

2. The body's natural sunscreen is:
   a) cytoplasm
   b) melanin
   c) adenosine triphosphate
   d) epithelial tissue

   b

3. The study of cells and cellular biology is called:
   a) histology
   b) pathology
   c) cytology
   d) cellology

   C

4. The structural unit (basic building block) of all living organisms is:
   a) a cell
   b) a tissue
   c) an organ
   d) a system

   a

5. The cell membrane provides the following to the cell:
   a) protection
   b) shape
   c) a structure that helps regulate the flow of materials going into and out of the cell
   d) all of the above are correct

   d

6. What is the main job of the cell?
   a) reproduction
   b) production of fats
   c) production of protein
   d) production of carbohydrates

   C

7. Protozoa are:
   a) one-celled organisms   c) nutrients
   b) multi-celled organisms   d) tissues

   a

8. The characteristic of letting some substances in and shutting out others is called:
   a) osmosis   c) homeostasis
   b) active transport   d) selective permeability

   d

9. The jelly-like liquid within the cell is called:
   a) protoplasm
   b) electrolyte
   c) cytoplasm
   d) physiological salt water solution

   c

10. The small structures that protrude out of the cell membrane and receive signals from other parts of the body are called:
    a) mitochondria   c) receptor sites
    b) amino acids   d) organelles

    c

11. Sacs that produce enzymes to break down large molecules of nutrients into smaller chemical structures are called:
    a) lysosomes   c) ribosomes
    b) vacuoles   d) chromosomes

    a

12. Special fibers made of nucleic acids and proteins are called:
    a) melanin   c) lysosomes
    b) chromatin   d) follicles

    b

13. Proteins are stored and later released from the cell by the:
    a) cell membrane   c) Golgi apparatus
    b) cytoplasm   d) nucleus

    c

14. Often referred to as the powerhouse of the cell, what supplies the cell with energy?
    a) Golgi apparatus   c) cell membranes
    b) ribosomes   d) mitochondria

    d

15. Cell division characterized by chromosome duplication and the formation of two identical daughter cells is known as:
    a) mitosis
    c) merkel cells
    b) meiosis
    d) DNA

    a

16. Which of the following characteristics is determined by the genes?
    a) blue eyes
    c) acne
    b) male pattern baldness
    d) all of the above are correct

    d

17. DNA is:
    a) dehydronucleic acid
    c) determined nucleic action
    b) deoxyribonucleic acid
    d) none of the above are correct

    b

18. Deoxyribonucleic acid:
    a) is exactly the same as ATP
    b) is located in the protoplasm of the cell
    c) carries genetic information
    d) is not involved with genes or chromosomes

    c

19. The nucleus of a cell is made primarily of:
    a) acids
    c) proteins
    b) ribosomes
    d) lysosomes

    c

20. The part of a cell that controls the activities of the cell is the:
    a) hair follicle
    c) mitochondria
    b) nucleus
    d) zygote

    b

21. The organelles responsible for the synthesis of protein are:
    a) Golgi apparatus
    c) lysosomes
    b) ribosomes
    d) mitochondria

    b

22. Which part of the human body has the greatest number of sweat glands?
    a) hands and feet
    c) the armpits
    b) the groin area
    d) scalp

    a

23. Cells that carry out different functions within the body are called:
    a) specialized cells
    c) diversified cells

b) tissues   d) mitochondria   *a*

24. The main function of a cell is to:
    a) produce protein
    b) produce hair
    c) divide into two identical daughter cells
    d) process oxygen   *a*

25. How does the skin regulate body temperature in the cold?
    a) through a decrease in blood flow
    b) through an increase in blood flow
    c) through production of sweat
    d) through production of sebum   *a*

26. Tissue found lining the inside of the body and its organs is:
    a) connective   c) endothelial
    b) striated   d) visceral   *c*

27. What is a tissue in human anatomy?
    a) a group of similar cells   c) membranes
    b) epithelium   d) matrix   *a*

28. Which of the following is NOT a type of muscle?
    a) visceral   c) striated
    b) lymph   d) cardiac   *b*

29. Striated muscle is:
    a) myocardial muscle   c) always involuntary
    b) skeletal   d) always voluntary   *b*

30. The important function of epithelial tissue is:
    a) to relay nerve impulses
    b) to serve as storage for fat
    c) to bear great amounts of weight in the body
    d) protection, absorption, and secretion   *d*

31. One of the principal locations of stratified squamous epithelium
    in the body is the:
    a) tubules of the kidney   c) epidermis of the skin
    b) fallopian tubes   d) brain   *c*

32. Tendons and ligaments derive much of their strength from the fact that they are composed of:
    a) hyaline cartilage
    b) bones
    c) skeletal muscle
    d) dense connective tissue

    d

33. The hair follicle is:
    a) a gland
    b) a cell
    c) a pore
    d) none of the above are correct

    c

34. Merkel cells are located:
    a) in the epidermis
    b) in the dermis
    c) in the papillary layer
    d) in the subcutis

    a

35. Which of the following structures is NOT an example of a tissue?
    a) cartilage
    b) bone
    c) heart
    d) epidermis

    c

36. The tissue specialized for movement is:
    a) epithelial
    b) muscular
    c) connective
    d) nervous

    b

37. Fat tissue is also called:
    a) endothelial tissue
    b) epithelial tissue
    c) adipose tissue
    d) connective tissue

    c

38. Tissue found lining the surfaces of organs is:
    a) cartilage
    b) connective
    c) epithelial
    d) muscular

    c

39. Which of the following is NOT a function of epithelial tissue?
    a) absorption
    b) protection
    c) contraction
    d) secretion

    c

40. The sweat glands in the armpits and groin are called:
    a) sebaceous glands
    b) apocrine glands
    c) endocrine glands
    d) helocrine glands

    b

41. Ligaments are made of:
    a) epithelial tissue
    b) reticular connective tissue
    c) fibrous connective tissue
    d) muscle tissue

    c

42. Lymph is a:

a) fat tissue
c) connective tissue
b) liquid tissue
d) none of the above are correct ___ *b*

43. Tissue which provides support and protection and binds structures together is:
a) epithelial
c) muscular
b) nervous
d) connective ___ *d*

44. Which of the following is NOT formed from connective tissue?
a) epidermis
c) cartilage
b) bones
d) adipose tissue ___ *a*

45. Which one of the following statements is correct?
a) Smooth muscles are attached to the bones to provide movement.
b) Smooth muscle contraction is involuntary.
c) The heart is made up of smooth muscle tissue.
d) Smooth muscles may be massive, like the trapezius. ___ *b*

46. Visceral muscles are also called:
a) voluntary muscles
c) smooth muscles
b) skeletal muscles
d) cardiac muscles ___ *c*

47. Which one of the following types of muscle is considered to be under voluntary nervous control?
a) cardiac
c) skeletal
b) visceral
d) smooth ___ *c*

48. In the epidermal layer of the skin, which one of the following is the layer containing fully keratinized epithelial cells?
a) stratum granulosum
c) stratum lucidum
b) stratum basale
d) stratum corneum ___ *d*

49. New cells of the skin are produced at the:
a) stratum corneum
c) stratum basale / germinativum
b) stratum granulosum
d) sebaceous gland ___ *c*

50. Keratinization of the epidermis starts in the:
a) stratum basale
c) stratum granulosum
b) stratum spinosum
d) stratum lucidum ___ *c*

51. Keratinocytes make up how much of the epidermis?

a) about 95%   c) about 75%
b) about 50%   d) about 25%   *a*

52. The cells which make the skin's pigment are called:
    a) keratinocytes   c) erythrocytes
    b) lymphocytes   d) melanocytes   *d*

53. Which of the following glands are attached to some hair follicles?
    a) eccrine   c) endocrine
    b) apocrine   d) exocrine   *b*

54. Skin is thickest on the:
    a) eyelids   c) back
    b) nose   d) hands   *c*

55. The prescription medication tretinoin is better known as:
    a) Reticulin   c) Retin-A
    b) elastin   d) hyaluronic acid   *c*

56. The bottom part of the hair that attaches to the papilla is called the:
    a) root   c) medulla
    b) bulb   d) matrix   *b*

57. Which of the following glands are attached to the hair follicle?
    a) eccrine sweat glands   c) pituitary gland
    b) sebaceous glands   d) thyroid gland   *b*

58. Another name for the basal layer of the epidermis is:
    a) stratum granulosum   c) stratum germinativum
    b) stratum spinosum   d) stratum basale   *c*

59. Collagen makes up how much of the total weight of the skin?
    a) 25%   c) 70%
    b) 50%   d) 90%   *c*

60. The skin regulates body temperature in hot weather by:
    a) reducing the amount of sweat
    b) producing more sebum

c) causing the erection of the arrector pili muscles
d) causing the dilation of blood vessels

d

61. The skin acts as a sensory organ because it contains:
    a) nerve endings   c) lymphatic vessels
    b) capillaries   d) sebaceous glands

a

62. The skin is able to register five different senses, which are:
    a) touch, pressure, sight, smell, and taste
    b) touch, pressure, smell, pain, and cold
    c) pain, cold, touch, pressure, and taste
    d) pain, cold, touch, pressure, and heat

d

63. Skin is thinnest on the:
    a) palms of the hands   c) neck
    b) cheeks   d) eyelids

d

64. Fibroblasts are responsible for:
    a) the movement of particles through a membrane
    b) the production of melanin
    c) the formation of collagen
    d) the engulfing of water by a cell

c

65. Macrophage cells and mast cells are:
    a) immune cells   c) keratinocytes
    b) collagen-producing cells   d) red blood cells

a

66. What are the functions of the skin?
    a) nourishing and breathing
    b) secretion and touch
    c) protection, temperature regulation, healing, immunity, sensation
    d) protection and sense of heat and cold

c

67. The two layers of the dermis are:
    a) basal layer and adipose layer
    b) papillary layer and reticular layer
    c) collagen layer and spiny layer
    d) fatty layer and elastin layer

b

68. What is ground substance?
    a) a substance that helps us ground the energy
    b) tretinoin

c) a keloid
d) fluid between the fibers in the dermis   *d*

69. What is a Meissner corpuscle?
    a) a piece of German china
    b) a nerve transmitter in the dermis
    c) an organelle in the cell, responsible for energy production
    d) a cell in the epidermis responsible for pigment production   *b*

70. Cell layers within the epidermis are known as epidermal:
    a) strada   c) strata
    b) striae   d) desmosomes   *c*

71. Which is NOT a type of striated muscle tissue?
    a) facial muscle   c) cardiac muscle
    b) skeletal muscle   d) visceral muscle   *d*

72. Which of these muscles is voluntary?
    a) cardiac muscle
    b) skeletal muscle
    c) smooth muscle
    d) none of the above are correct   *b*

73. Which of these are responsible for smiling?
    a) skeletal muscle in the face
    b) smooth muscles in the face
    c) tendons in the face
    d) ligaments in the face   *a*

74. Bone is attached to bone by:
    a) fascia   c) aponeurosis
    b) ligaments   d) tendons   *b*

75. A narrow band of fibrous tissue that attaches a muscle to a bone
    is called:
    a) aponeurosis   c) ligament
    b) fascia   d) tendon   *d*

Chapter **3**

BODY SYSTEMS

1. How many systems are there in the human body?
   a) 3   c) 7
   b) 6   d) 10   _____

2. The system used to pump blood around the body is the:
   a) cardiovascular system   c) respiratory system
   b) immune system   d) urinary system   _____

3. Which system transports gases to and from body tissue and supplies fresh oxygen?
   a) the skeletal system   c) the cardiovascular system
   b) the respiratory system   d) the urinary system   _____

4. Which of these systems does NOT influence waste removal?
   a) the urinary system   c) the digestive system
   b) the cardiovascular system d) none of the above
                                    are correct   _____

5. This system can be removed without endangering human life:
   a) the endocrine system   c) the digestive system
   b) the immune system   d) the reproductive system   _____

6. Half of the body's bulk is from:
   a) the muscular system   c) the nervous system
   b) the skeletal system   d) water   _____

7. The basis of consciousness is in the:
   a) heart   c) spinal cord
   b) lungs   d) brain   _____

8. Support, protection of soft tissue, mineral storage, and blood formation are functions of which system?
   a) the muscular system
   b) the skeletal system
   c) the nervous system
   d) the circulatory system   _____

9. Which system directs long-term changes in the activities of other organ systems?
   a) the nervous system
   b) the reproductive system
   c) the endocrine system
   d) the immune system   _____

10. Production of waste is influenced by:
    a) blood flow
    b) the endocrine system
    c) normal body rhythms and cycles
    d) all of the above are correct   _____

11. The endocrine system regulates:
    a) the stomach and intestines
    b) the kidneys
    c) the reproductive organs
    d) all of the above are correct   _____

12. An antibody would be produced in which system?
    a) the endocrine system
    b) the immune system
    c) the digestive system
    d) the urinary system   _____

13. Functions regulated by hormones include:
    a) metabolism
    b) growth and sexual development
    c) water and mineral balance
    d) all of the above are correct   _____

14. An example of an androgen is:
    a) estrogen
    b) testosterone
    c) progesterone
    d) none of the above are correct   _____

15. Acne can be caused by:
    a) excessive androgens
    b) underproduction of progesterone
    c) a and b are correct
    d) neither a nor b is correct   _____

16. Progesterone can benefit the skin in which way(s)?
    a) by supporting the production of important moisture binders such as hyalronic acid
    b) by helping to foster cellular turnover
    c) a and b are correct
    d) neither a nor b is correct   _____

17. The size and activity of the sebaceous gland in the pore is regulated by:
    a) estrogen   c) testosterone
    b) progesterone   d) androgens   _____

18. Dry, itchy skin and hair breakage can be a result of:
    a) overproduction of steroids
    b) underproduction of steroids
    c) underproduction of thyroid hormone
    d) overproduction of thyroid hormone   _____

19. The adrenal glands can be found:
    a) just below the kidneys
    b) on top of the kidneys
    c) on both sides of the kidneys
    d) none of the above are correct   _____

20. This gland is responsible for the beginning of the immune system in young persons:
    a) the thymus gland   c) the pancreas
    b) the thyroid gland   d) the tonsils   _____

21. Blood completes a full circuit of the body in about:
    a) 30 seconds   c) five minutes
    b) one minute   d) fifteen minutes   _____

22. A thick-walled, elastic vessel through which oxygenated blood is pumped throughout the body is a:
    a) capillary   c) artery
    b) vein   d) none of the above
                                            are correct   _____

23. Venous capillaries carry:
    a) oxygenated blood to the heart
    b) deoxygenated blood to the heart
    c) oxygenated blood from the heart
    d) deoxygenated blood away from the heart   _____

24. The main artery that supplies the head and face is the:
    a) aorta
    c) superior temporal artery
    b) carotid
    d) superior vena cava   _____

25. The clear part of the liquid is called serum or:
    a) platelets
    c) red blood cells
    b) leukocytes
    d) plasma   _____

26. Which of these statements is false?
    a) Lymph is colorless, like plasma.
    b) Lymph flows in both directions, like blood.
    c) Lymph flows towards the heart.
    d) Lymph bathes tissues and removes wastes and foreign bodies.   _____

27. Lymph nodes can be found everywhere in concentrated nodes in:
    a) the chest
    c) the neck
    b) the groin
    d) all of the above are correct   _____

28. MLD (Manual Lymph Drainage) may be performed for all of the
    following except:
    a) acne
    c) swelling
    b) malignant tumors
    d) facelift preparation   _____

29. An antigen can be:
    a) a virus
    c) T-helper cells
    b) Langerhans cells
    d) none of the above
       are correct   _____

30. Histamine is secreted by which cells?
    a) mast cells
    c) macrophage cells
    b) T-killer cells
    d) T-helper cells   _____

31. An example of an autoimmune disease is:
    a) lupus
    c) hives
    b) diabetes
    d) obesity   _____

32. Which of these systems lies only within the circulatory system?
    a) the nervous system
    c) the urinary system
    b) the muscular system
    d) the lymphatic system   _____

Chapter 4

BONES, MUSCLES, AND NERVES OF THE FACE AND SKULL

1. Knowledge of the skin structure is important when:
   a) administering massage technique
   b) operating facial machines for muscle lifting
   c) performing hair removal by waxing
   d) designing corrective makeup   _____

2. How many bones are in the human body?
   a) 206   c) 266
   b) 235   d) it varies according to age   _____

3. Bones are:
   a) 1/3 organic, 2/3 inorganic   c) all organic
   b) 2/3 organic and 1/3 inorganic d) all inorganic   _____

4. Inorganic means:
   a) relating to an organ
   b) composed of matter related to living tissue
   c) composed of matter not related to living organisms
   d) made up of fibrous tissue   _____

5. Bones:
   a) protect organs against injury
   b) serve as attachments for muscles
   c) a and b are correct
   d) neither a nor b is correct   _____

6. The cranium contains:
   a) 8 bones   c) 22 bones
   b) 14 bones   d) 206 bones   _____

7. How many bones are in the skull?
   a) 8   c) 22
   b) 14   d) 1   _____

8. Which of these is NOT a cranial bone?
   a) the frontal bone   c) the ethmoid bones
   b) the sphenoid   d) the temporal bones   _____

9. Which are NOT facial bones?
   a) the temporal bones   c) the nasal bones
   b) the ethmoid bones   d) the zygomatic bones _____

10. Which bone or bones are NOT situated near the mouth?
    a) the palatine bones   c) the occipital bone
    b) the maxillae   d) the mandible   _____

11. The lacrimal bones are:
    a) light spongy bones between the eyesockets
    b) the sockets of the eyes
    c) at the top of the nose and form the nose bridge
    d) also called the cheekbones   _____

12. The technical name for the Adam's apple is:
    a) the sphenoid   c) the hyoid
    b) the ethmoid bones   d) the cranial vault   _____

13. The parietal bones are:
    a) bones of the face   c) bone of the neck
    b) bones of the cranium   d) bones of the hand   _____

14. Muscles comprise about how much of body weight?
    a) 15%   c) 44%
    b) 32%   d) 70%   _____

15. Facial muscles are not:
    a) voluntary muscles
    b) made of contractile fibrous tissue
    c) contracted by a physiochemical reaction
    d) layered   _____

16. Muscles are made of protein structures known as:
    a) mitochondria   c) synapses
    b) myofibrils   d) the aponeurosis   _____

17. The end of the muscle attached to the stationary bone is the:
    a) origin   c) belly
    b) insertion   d) none of the above
                                are correct   _____

18. Pronators are found:
    a) in the shoulders   c) in the forearms
    b) in the neck region   d) in the area of the eyebrows _____

19. Botox treatments for removing frown lines on the forehead will
    be injected into the:
    a) obicularis oculi   c) temporalis
    b) obicularis oris   d) corrugator   _____

20. Which muscle is chiefly responsible for chewing?
    a) masseter   c) zygomatic minor
    b) zygomatic major   d) mandible   _____

21. The muscle responsible for a firm chin and neck is:
    a) cervical vertebrae   c) platysma
    b) sternocleidomastoid   d) hyoid   _____

22. Which muscles do NOT achieve movement of the shoulders?
    a) trapezius and latissimus dorsi
    b) biceps
    c) the pectoralis
    d) serratus anterior   _____

23. How many muscles are in the human body?
    a) over 500   c) 200
    b) 100   d) 1,000   _____

24. The central part of the muscle is the:
    a) core   c) origin
    b) belly   d) insertion area   _____

25. The mandible is:
    a) the upper jaw
    b) the lower jawbone
    c) the frontal bone
    d) the Adam's apple   _____

26. The facial muscles are situated below which layer of the skin?
    a) the epidermis
    b) the dermis
    c) the subcutaneous layer
    d) none of the above are correct   _____

27. Bone tissue contains:
    a) blood vessels
    b) nerves
    c) minerals
    d) all of the above are correct   _____

28. The largest mass of nerve tissue:
    a) are the genitals
    b) is the brain
    c) is the spinal cord
    d) are the lips   _____

29. The spinal cord consists of how many pairs of spinal nerves?
    a) 30
    b) 31
    c) 32
    d) 33   _____

30. How many pairs of cranial nerves originate in the brain?
    a) 8
    b) 12
    c) 14
    d) 22   _____

31. The main sensory nerve of the face is the:
    a) 1st cranial nerve
    b) 5th cranial nerve
    c) 7th nerve
    d) 12th nerve   _____

32. Motor nerves extend from the main facial motor nerve, which is the:
    a) 1st cranial nerve
    b) 5th nerve
    c) 7th nerve
    d) 12th nerve   _____

33. Which of these is NOT part of the 5th cranial nerve?
    a) the mandibular nerve
    b) the maxillary nerve
    c) the ophthalmic nerve
    d) the temporal nerve   _____

34. Relaxation is induced by stimulating a(n):
    a) synapse
    b) reflex action
    c) motor point
    d) afferent neuron   _____

Chapter *5*

BACTERIOLOGY AND SANITATION

1. Which of these is NOT a microorganism?
   - a) airborne germs
   - b) pathogenic bacteria
   - c) host cells
   - d) yeast

   _____

2. Infection and disease are likely with all except:
   - a) nonpathogenic bacteria
   - b) spirilla
   - c) fungi
   - d) cocci

   _____

3. Sterilization kills:
   - a) good bacteria
   - b) hepatitis virus
   - c) fungal spores
   - d) all of the above are correct

   _____

4. Autoclaves:
   - a) sterilize and kill all microorganisms
   - b) disinfect in a special chamber that uses high heat and pressure
   - c) are antiseptics designed for use on human skin
   - d) are wet sanitizing agents

   _____

5. Which would you NOT autoclave?
   - a) electrolysis needle
   - b) sponges
   - c) comedone extractor
   - d) glass electrodes

   _____

6. Hydrogen peroxide is an example of:
   - a) a wet sanitizing agent
   - b) a hospital grade disinfectant
   - c) an antiseptic
   - d) a sterilizer

   _____

7. Items that can NOT be disposed in a covered trash receptacle are:
   a) tongue depressors
   b) lancets
   c) esthetician's gloves
   d) none of the above are correct _____

8. A sharps box is NOT used for:
   a) disposing of lancets
   b) preventing injury from contaminated items
   c) machine attachments
   d) needles _____

9. Disposable items include:
   a) headbands
   b) machine attachments
   c) latex or vinyl gloves
   d) mask brushes _____

10. Which is NOT a blood-borne pathogen?
    a) herpes simplex
    b) HIV
    c) tuberculosis
    d) hepatitis _____

11. The process of properly handling sterilized or disinfected equipment so it does not become contaminated by microorganisms before being used by a client is:
    a) cross-contamination procedure
    b) contamination procedure
    c) autoclaving procedure
    d) aseptic procedure _____

12. The agency that oversees workplace safety for employees is the:
    a) FDA
    b) Cosmetics, Toiletry, and Fragrance Association (CTFA)
    c) Cosmetology Commission
    d) Occupational Safety and Health Administration _____

13. A Materials Safety Data Sheet is NOT required for:
    a) nail chemicals
    b) germicides
    c) harmless skin-care products
    d) machines and attachments safety _____

14. Which of these is NOT included in the Materials Safety Data Sheet?
    a) how to handle spills
    b) flammability
    c) quantity in storage
    d) toxicity _____

15. The Occupational Safety and Health Administration (OSHA) can NOT:
    a) set regulations for safety in the workplace
    b) conduct unannounced inspection of employers
    c) condemn skin-care products based on ineffective results
    d) enforce fines for consuming food in the salon work area _____

16. Objects that have no live microorganisms present on them are described as:
    a) sterile
    b) antiseptic
    c) aseptic
    d) none of the above are correct_____

17. Disinfectants designed for use in human skin are:
    a) aseptics
    b) sanitizers
    c) sterilizers
    d) antiseptics _____

18. Athlete's foot is an example of:
    a) algae
    b) fungus
    c) virus
    d) bacteria _____

19. Mycoses are:
    a) algae-related infections
    b) fungus-related infections
    c) virus-related infections
    d) bacteria-related infections _____

20. Which of the following is NOT a disinfectant chemical?
    a) glutaraldehyde
    b) benzalkonium chloride
    c) tertiary ammonium compounds
    d) isopropyl alcohol _____

Chapter 6

NUTRITION

1. When broken down into basic molecules, food is used by the cells to:
   a) repair damage
   b) form new cells
   c) conduct the biochemical reactions that run the body's systems
   d) all of the above are correct

   D

2. What is responsible for moving nutrients around the body and into cells?
   a) water
   b) proteins
   c) fiber
   d) carbohydrates

   A

3. Dietary sources of protein include:
   a) glucose
   b) apples
   c) beans
   d) bananas

   C

4. Which of these is NOT a basic building block or nutrient?
   a) fat
   b) fiber
   c) carbohydrates
   d) proteins

   B

5. Which is NOT one of protein's functions?
   a) to make other usable proteins
   b) to duplicate DNA
   c) to make muscle tissue, blood, and enzymes
   d) to be the main ingredient in blood, sweat, and other body fluids

   D

6. Why must essential amino acids be part of one's diet?
   a) the body makes them from other bodily chemicals
   b) the body cannot manufacture them
   c) the acids form chains to create fiber
   d) the acids form chains to create carbohydrates

   B

7. An adult body is made up of approximately:
   a) 44% water
   b) 60% water
   c) 75% water
   d) 90% water

   B

8. Fiber is made of an undigestible carbohydrate called:
   a) sucrose
   b) complex
   c) cellulose
   d) lactose

   C

9. What is the one-unit sugar molecule that all cells use for energy?
   a) disaccharide
   b) triglyceride
   c) polysaccaride
   d) monosaccharide

   D

10. Which is NOT true of linoleic acids?
    a) it attaches to carbon atoms
    b) it makes important hormones called prostaglandins
    c) it is not made by the body and must be taken in the diet
    d) it is found in oils made from safflower, corn, soybean, and sunflower

    A

11. Vegans stick to diets of:
    a) plants only
    b) plants and dairy, but no meat
    c) plants and fish for protein, but no dairy or meat
    d) high protein and low carbohydrates

    A

12. How does the caloric content of a gram of fat compare to the caloric content of a gram of carbohydrate or protein?
    a) A gram of fat has 4 calories; a gram of carbohydrate or protein has 4 calories.
    b) A gram of fat or a gram of protein has 9 calories; a gram of carbohydrate has 4 calories.
    c) A gram of fat or a gram of carbohydrate has 9 calories; a gram of protein has 4 calories.
    d) A gram of fat has 9 calories; a gram of carbohydrate or protein has 4 calories.

    D

13. These are all carbohydrates except:
    a) lactose
    b) starch
    c) cellulose
    d) lipids

    D

14. What is produced when polyunsaturated oil is partially hydrogenated?
    a) omega-3 fatty acids
    c) polysaccharides
    b) trans fatty acids
    d) prostaglandin

    B

15. What is NOT true of vitamins?
    a) many are involved in energy release from carbohydrates
    b) they can be synthesized by the body
    c) they are required for synthesizing fatty acids
    d) they are required for breaking down and constructing proteins

    B

16. Vitamin A is needed for:
    a) growth and repair of body tissue
    b) health in hair, skin, and nails
    c) red blood cell formation
    d) regulation of liver, kidneys, and gall bladder

    A

17. Which of these vitamins is called the sunshine vitamin?
    a) vitamin A
    c) vitamin D
    b) vitamin C
    d) vitamin E

    C

18. A glucose molecule is also known as a(n):
    a) essential amino acid
    c) monosaccharide
    b) glucagon
    d) none of the above are correct

    C

19. An example of a digestible polysaccharide is:
    a) fruit sugar
    c) fiber
    b) starch
    d) sucrose

    B

20. Lactose is a:
    a) monosaccharide
    c) polysaccharide
    b) disaccharide
    d) lipid

    B

21. Lipids are NOT used for:
    a) making hormones
    c) the absorption of vitamin B
    b) creating cell membranes
    d) a source of energy

    C

22. The main fat in foods are:
    a) polysaccharides
    c) polyunsaturated fatty acids
    b) monounsaturated fatty acids
    d) triglycerides

    D

23. Unsaturated fatty acids are made up of atoms of:
    a) hydrogen
    b) amino acids
    c) triglycerides
    d) carbon

    D

24. A gram of fat has:
    a) 4 calories
    b) 6 calories
    c) 8 calories
    d) 9 calories

    D

25. It takes the body about how many extra calories to store a pound of fat?
    a) 1000
    b) 1500
    c) 2500
    d) 3500

    D

26. Cholesterol will NOT be found in:
    a) eggs
    b) shrimp
    c) fish
    d) soy

    D

27. Which fish is recommended as being highest in omega 3 fatty acids?
    a) tuna
    b) trout
    c) salmon
    d) shark

    C

28. Betacarotene is NOT:
    a) a provitamin
    b) a precursor
    c) water soluble
    d) found in spinach

    C

29. Vitamin E is also known as:
    a) thiamine
    b) tocopheral
    c) retinoid
    d) pellagra

    B

30. Vitamin B-2 will alleviate:
    a) elevated cholesterol
    b) cracks and lesions in the corner of the mouth
    c) dermatitis
    d) osteoporosis and poor bone growth

    B

31. What vitamin is responsible for collagen maintenance?
    a) K
    b) chromium
    c) ascorbic acid
    d) F

    C

32. Zinc can be found in:
    a) fish eggs, nuts, cabbage
    b) bananas
    c) dairy products
    d) whole grains, wheat bran

    D

33. What is an example of provitamin A?
    a) adipose
    b) betacarotene
    c) retinol
    d) precursor

    B

34. A vitamin A deficiency may result in:
    a) night blindness
    b) improper maintenance of epithelial tissue
    c) follicular keratinosis
    d) all of the above are correct

    D

35. What is NOT true of betacarotene?
    a) it helps control free radicals
    b) it may play a role in the formation of immune system cells
    c) it is responsible for the bright color of fruits and vegetables
    d) it enables the body to absorb calcium

    D

36. Vitamin D is called the sunshine vitamin because:
    a) the skin synthesizes vitamin D from cholesterol when exposed to sunlight
    b) it is obtained from eating egg yolks and butter
    c) it is found in bright vegetables
    d) it is used to treat sun-damaged skin

    A

37. Because it is an antioxidant, vitamin E (also called tocopherol):
    a) is used to treat follicular keratinosis
    b) is a contributing cause of osteoperosis
    c) cannot be stored in body fat
    d) can protect the body from damage caused by free radicals

    D

38. What is true of vitamin K?
    a) it is found in pork, beef, and fortified cereals
    b) it is responsible for the synthesis factors necessary for blood coagulation
    c) a vitamin K deficiency is common
    d) a deficiency of vitamin K is called pellegra

    B

39. Which water-soluble vitamin is required for the manufacture of steroids?
    a) riboflavin
    b) thiamine
    c) niacin
    d) pyridoxine

    C

40. What disorder is caused by a lack of vitamin B12?
    a) pellagra
    b) pernicious anemia
    c) hard-to-control bleeding
    d) beriberi

    B

41. Which element is necessary to properly transport oxygen to cells?
    a) zinc
    b) copper
    c) iron
    d) selenium

42. A good diet includes these percentages of basic foods:
    a) 15-20% fat, 30% protein, 55-60% carbohydrates
    b) 15-20% fat, 30% carbohydrates, 55-60% protein
    c) 15-20% carbohydrates, 30% fat, 55-60% protein
    d) 15-20% protein, 30% fat, 55-60% carbohydrates

43. What is NOT true of weight loss?
    a) vitamins and supplements may substitute for proper nutrition
    b) certain diets may cause chemical imbalances
    c) the best way to lose weight is a healthy diet and proper exercise
    d) vitamins and minerals do not have much effect without macronutrients

Chapter 7

ROOM FURNISHINGS

1. The most important piece of equipment in a treatment room is the:
   a) esthetic chair
   b) operator stool
   c) step stool
   d) utility cart

   a

2. A hydraulic motorized bed:
   a) can be used without needing an energy supply
   b) should never be used for both facials and massage
   c) can be arranged in several different positions to elevate different areas
   d) all of the above are correct

   c

3. An ergonomically correct stool:
   a) is designed to blend in with treatment rooms, hospitals, or offices
   b) often does not have a back rest
   c) is practically designed in sturdy, nonporous fabric
   d) is healthy for the human spine

   d

4. When in doubt, clean equipment and tools with:
   a) ammonia
   b) window cleaner
   c) scouring powder
   d) mild soap and water

   d

5. To avoid back problems and tension buildup:
   a) have the client's head at your collar bone
   b) keep your hands at a 45-degree angle during the facial massage
   c) rest your elbows on the bed near the client's ears
   d) all of the above are correct

   c

6. Estheticians should:
   a) take breaks only if not fully booked for the day
   b) drink plenty of soft drinks
   c) avoid going outside between treatments
   d) rotate and perform hand exercises

7. Back bar items are NOT:
   a) relevant retail products displayed for the client's benefit
   b) sometimes stored in the treatment room
   c) organized on a trolley in most spas
   d) pumped out from the dispensary in some spas, as each client arrives

Chapter 8

TECHNOLOGICAL TOOLS

1. A magnifying lamp measures its power in:
   a) hertz
   b) diopters
   c) volts
   d) watts

   B

2. A 5 diopter lamp has:
   a) 5 x power magnification
   b) 50 x power magnification
   c) 500 x power magnification
   d) none of the above are correct

   B

3. Maintenance on the lamp includes:
   a) tightening the arm
   b) periodically unscrewing the light
   c) a and b are correct
   d) neither a nor b is correct

   A

4. What color is the filtered light used in a Wood's lamp?
   a) bright white
   b) fluorescent
   c) infrared
   d) black

   D

5. The Wood's lamp allows the esthetician to:
   a) diagnose a disease
   b) analyze thin skin
   c) a and b are correct
   d) neither a nor b is correct

   B

6. When using the Wood's lamp, avoid:
   a) looking into the lamp
   b) touching the skin
   c) using any other lighting in the room
   d) all of the above are correct

   D

7. The skin scope analyzer uses a(n):
   a) bright white light
   b) fluorescent white light
   c) infrared light
   d) deep violet light

   D

8. A skin scope's rays can penetrate up to:
   a) the corneum layer
   b) the granular layer
   c) the basal layer
   d) the reticulary dermis

   C

9. Under the Wood's Lamp and the skin scope, the color yellow depicts:
   a) sun damage
   b) dehydrated skin
   c) normal healthy skin
   d) comedones

   D

10. Bright fluorescent under the Wood's lamp and the skin scope depicts:
    a) dehydrated skin
    b) normal healthy skin
    c) hydrated skin
    d) sun damage

    C

11. A thick cornea layer shows up under the Wood's lamp as:
    a) white fluorescent
    b) white spots
    c) blue-white
    d) brown

    A

12. When using the rotary brush for oily skin:
    a) use slow, steady rotations
    b) apply extra pressure
    c) place the brush at a 45-degree angle
    d) none of the above are correct

    D

13. Rotary brushes must be:
    a) clean and dry when being used
    b) avoided on acne or inflamed skin
    c) used starting at the jawbone
    d) none of the above are correct

    B

14. The vacuum machine does all except:
    a) suction dirt and impurities out of the skin
    b) stimulate blood circulation
    c) reduce the appearance of creases
    d) reduce broken capillaries

    D

15. Steamers are useful for:
    a) softening sebum and debris
    b) oxygenating the skin
    c) antiseptic qualities
    d) all of the above are correct

    D

16. Air is made up of approximately:
    a) 20% oxygen   c) 55% oxygen
    b) 45% oxygen   d) 85% oxygen

    A

17. Ozone, as found in a steamer, is represented according to its composition as:
    a) O_2 c) H_2O_2
    b) O_3 d) H_3O

    B

18. When using a steamer, always:
    a) place mineral water in the designated container
    b) switch the ozone on right away to test for steam
    c) place the steamer 6 inches away from the client
    d) none of the above are correct

    D

19. About how far must the steamer be from the face of a client with normal skin?
    a) 6 inches   c) 24 inches
    b) 15 inches   d) as close as the client requests

    B

20. An overabundance of steam:
    a) rehydrates the skin   c) a and b are correct
    b) irritates the skin   d) neither a nor b is correct

    B

21. Which of these can cause potential damage?
    a) topping off the steamer with cool water while in service
    b) creating aromatherapy through adding essential oils to the water
    c) filling the container above the designated level
    d) all of the above are correct

    D

22. Clients can be burned from a steamer if:
    a) there are mineral deposits in the jar
    b) you pour water above the maximum level
    c) a and b are correct
    d) neither a nor b is correct

    C

23. When cleaning a steamer, never:
    a) use white vinegar
    b) turn the steamer on
    c) allow the steamer to soak overnight
    d) keep the ozone off

    C

24. The Lucas spray is particularly beneficial to:
    a) couperose skin
    b) thick skin
    c) oily skin
    d) none of the above are correct_____ A

25. High frequency has the ability to change polarity:
    a) 100 times per second
    b) 5,000 times per second
    c) 60,000 to 200,000 times per second
    d) 1,000,000 times per second _____ C

26. The galvanic machine:
    a) has an antiseptic effect on the skin
    b) helps to coagulate and heal any open lesion in the skin
    c) converts oscillating current from an outlet into direct current
    d) causes water vibration in the skin _____ C

27. The high frequency machine:
    a) uses Tesla Pulse Train current
    b) uses sinusoidal current
    c) a and b are correct
    d) neither a nor b is correct _____ C

28. The blue or violet light in the high frequency electrode comes from:
    a) infrared rays
    b) ultraviolet rays
    c) neon gas
    d) argon gas _____ D

29. The red, pink, or orange light emitted from the high frequency electrode comes from:
    a) infrared rays
    b) ultraviolet rays
    c) neon gas
    d) argon gas _____ C

30. With the spiral indirect high frequency:
    a) the client holds the glass electrode
    b) oily and problem skin benefits most
    c) contact with the skin can be broken, since it is indirect current
    d) all of the above are correct _____ A

31. Electrodes can be cleaned by:
    a) soaking the electrode in a gentle solution for 20 minutes
    b) sterilization in a UV machine
    c) a and b are correct
    d) neither a nor b is correct _____ D

32. Disincrustation is best for:
    a) oily skin
    b) sagging skin
    c) rosacea
    d) mature skin _____ A

33. Galvanic current achieves:
    a) chemical reactions in the skin   c) a and b are correct
    b) ionic reactions in the skin   d) neither a nor b is correct

    C

34. The chemical reaction that occurs when current transforms sebum into soap is:
    a) saponification, which occurs during disincrustation
    b) anaphoresis
    c) cataphoresis
    d) none of the above are correct

    A

35. Disincrustation is used on the:
    a) dryer areas of the skin   c) neck
    b) eyelids   d) none of the above are correct

    D

36. In disincrustation:
    a) the esthetician holds the positive electrode
    b) the positive electrode is connected to the red wire
    c) you should start with the switch on positive and use negative last
    d) all of the above are correct

    B

37. Iontophoresis means:
    a) introduction of ions
    b) penetrating moisture
    c) causing a chemical reaction
    d) something is based on the laws of attraction

    A

38. The positive pole causes:
    a) an acid reaction   c) increased blood circulation
    b) stimulated nerve endings   d) all of the above are correct

    A

39. The negative pole causes:
    a) an alkaline reaction   c) increased blood circulation
    b) stimulated nerve endings   d) all of the above are correct

    D

40. Calming and soothing nerve endings is achieved with the:
    a) positive pole in iontophoresis
    b) negative pole in iontophoresis
    c) positive pole in disincrustation
    d) negative pole in disncrustation

    A

41. Decreased blood circulation is achieved with the:
    a) positive pole in iontophoresis
    b) negative pole in iontophoresis
    c) positive pole in disincrustation
    d) negative pole in disincrustation

    A

42. If an ampoule's polarity is NOT indicated by the manufacturer in iontophoresis, always:
    a) use it on positive for 3-5 minutes, then negative for 3-5 minutes
    b) use it 3-5 minutes on positive only
    c) use it 3-5 minutes on negative, then 3-5 minutes on positive
    d) leave it alone, and explain professionally that you may not do this treatment

    C

43. The word cataphoresis refers to:
    a) by means of galvanic current   c) by means of high frequency
    b) by means of Tesla current   d) none of the above
                                             are correct

    D

44. The infusion of a negative product is:
    a) cataphoresis   c) iontophoresis
    b) anaphoresis   d) none of the above
                          are correct

    B

45. The negative pole in iontophoresis is called the:
    a) anode   c) electrode
    b) cathode   d) none of the above
                    are correct

    B

46. The ionto mask is used for:
    a) disincrustation   c) a and b are correct
    b) ionization   d) neither a nor b is correct

    C

47. When using the ionto mask:
    a) clients do not hold electrodes
    b) galvanic current is applied
    c) the client has a wet pad put under her shoulder
    d) all of the above are correct

    D

48. Microcurrent stimulation is used nowadays to treat conditions including:
    a) stroke and paralysis   c) Bells Palsy
    b) ligament injuries   d) all of the above are correct

    D

49. Which of these is NOT true for microcurrent?
    a) it can stretch out cramped and shortened muscles
    b) it stimulates collagen and elastin fibers
    c) it creates a natural tan on the skin
    d) all of the above are correct

    C

50. Current intensity has shapes such as:
    a) squares
    b) ramps
    c) sine waves
    d) all of the above are correct

    D

51. The mildest waveform is the:
    a) square wave
    b) circular wave
    c) rectangular wave
    d) sine wave

    D

52. Which wave type is referred to as a sharp form, due to its rapid rise and sharp drop-off?
    a) ramp
    b) square
    c) sine
    d) rectangular

    D

53. A current generator is known to:
    a) generate the bioelectric current flowing in the body
    b) cause muscles to contract completely
    c) regulate the current according to the skin's resistance
    d) all of the above are correct

    C

54. When using paraffin wax heaters, never:
    a) use heated paraffin for the face
    b) leave heated paraffin heaters on overnight
    c) use a substitute heater such as a crock pot for heating
    d) all of the above

    C

55. When using a hot towel cabbie, never:
    a) leave the door open at night
    b) clean inside by spraying 70% alcohol
    c) clean the ultraviolet lamps
    d) leave unused hot towels for the next day

    D

56. The heat mask uses:
    a) infrared heat
    b) ultraviolet heat
    c) solar heat
    d) none of the above are correct

    A

57. The heat mask works well with:
    a) the steamer
    b) hot towels
    c) a and b are correct
    d) neither a nor b is correct

    D

58. The heat mask should be kept on for:
    a) 5 minutes
    b) 10 minutes
    c) 15 minutes
    d) The particular treatment will dictate the appropriateness
    of the time.

    D

59. Boots and mitts are called add-on services, since:
    a) they are supplemented in otherwise complete treatments
    b) they were only added on the menu after the initial menu was completed
    c) they are added on the hands and feet
    d) none of the above are correct

    A

60. In microdermabrasion, crystals are made of corundum powder or:
    a) aluminum dioxide
    b) titanium dioxide
    c) zinc oxide
    d) none of the above are correct

    A

61. Microdermabrasion is used for:
    a) wrinkles and fine lines
    b) enlarged pores
    c) open and closed comedones
    d) all of the above are correct

    D

62. Microdermabrason is NOT recommended for:
    a) open and closed comedones
    b) inflammatory acne
    c) sun-damaged skin
    d) wrinkles

    B

63. Lasers used in medicine are fundamentally:
    a) an energy source
    b) microcrystals that can resurface burn and shine light
    c) bioelectrical signals used to correct a disorder
    d) none of the above are correct

    A

64. Which of these is true about lasers?
    a) they can cause a nuclear reaction
    b) they can "burn off" the top layer of the skin without touching
    the lower layer
    c) a and b are correct
    d) neither a nor b is correct

    C

Chapter 9

BASICS OF ELECTRICITY

1. What is responsible for holding together all atoms and molecules?
   - a) matter
   - b) chemical electrical signals
   - c) electric fields
   - d) electromagnestism
   _____

2. Electricity is used in medicine in:
   - a) photo light
   - b) electron microscopes
   - c) a and b are correct
   - d) neither a nor b is correct
   _____

3. A Magnetic Resonance Imager (MRI) allows doctors to:
   - a) test for possible cancerous cells
   - b) look inside the body without surgery
   - c) record tiny electrical signals from the heart
   - d) all of the above are correct
   _____

4. Electric stimulators can:
   - a) aid in healing muscles
   - b) eliminate spider veins
   - c) remove hair
   - d) none of the above are correct
   _____

5. Atoms are made up solely of:
   - a) electrons and protons
   - b) protons and neutrons
   - c) electrons and quarks
   - d) protons and quarks
   _____

6. Quarks make up larger particles called:
   - a) electrons
   - b) protons
   - c) electrons and neutrons
   - d) protons and neutrons
   _____

7. The nucleus comprises:
   a) atoms of electricity
   b) protons and neutrons
   c) electrons and protons
   d) electrons only   _____

8. Which of these is NOT electrically charged?
   a) electrons
   b) neutrons
   c) protons
   d) quarks   _____

9. A state of equilibrium exists when:
   a) the number of protons equals the number of neutrons
   b) the number of protons equals the number of electrons
   c) the number of neutrons equals the number of electrons
   d) the number of electrons equals the number of quarks
      in the nucleus   _____

10. A neutral atom:
    a) has the same number of protons and neutrons
    b) has more neutrons
    c) is negatively charged
    d) is in a state of equilibrium   _____

11. An example of a neutral atom is:
    a) hydrogen
    b) water
    c) an electrical conductor
    d) a sodium ion   _____

12. Which of these shows size increasing from smallest to largest?
    a) atom, element, matter
    b) element, atom, matter
    c) matter, element, atom
    d) none of the above are correct   _____

13. The innermost shell of an atom can have up to:
    a) 1 electron
    b) 2 electrons
    c) 4 electrons
    d) 8 electrons   _____

14. The 3rd shell can have up to:
    a) 2 electrons
    b) 8 electrons
    c) 18 electrons
    d) any amount, as long as it is equal to the number of protons   _____

15. The valence shell is the:
    - a) innermost shell
    - b) the 2nd shell
    - c) most stable shell
    - d) the outer axis   _____

16. Bound electrons are found in the:
    - a) neutral atom
    - b) valence shell
    - c) nucleus
    - d) the innermost shell   _____

17. Free electrons are found in the:
    - a) neutral atom
    - b) valence shell
    - c) nucleus
    - d) the innermost shell   _____

18. An imbalanced atom:
    - a) has taken on a negative charge
    - b) has taken on a positive charge
    - c) does not carry an electrical charge
    - d) is called an ion when it carries any charge   _____

19. When two or more atoms are locked together, what is formed?
    - a) an ion
    - b) a covalent bond
    - c) a molecule
    - d) ionic bonding   _____

20. A covalent bond involves:
    - a) giving away electrons to become stable
    - b) taking away electrons to become stable
    - c) two or more atoms sharing electrons
    - d) all of the above are correct   _____

21. The conductivity of a substance is determined by its:
    - a) valence shell
    - b) electrical charge
    - c) electric field
    - d) electromagnetism   _____

22. A lack of electrons on a surface will give that surface a:
    - a) negative charge
    - b) neutral charge
    - c) positive charge
    - d) none of the above are correct   _____

23. Electric fields are found:
    - a) in the nucleus of the atom
    - b) in the valence shell
    - c) around each atomic structure
    - d) in large fields close to power plants   _____

24. Which material structure is a good conductor?
    a) one with 5 electrons in its valence shell
    b) one with one electron in its outmost shell
    c) one in which the electrons are firmly bound
    d) one with a full valence shell   _____

25. An example of an insulator is:
    a) mercury   c) foil
    b) glass   d) electrode   _____

26. Copper is a good conductor since it:
    a) has a full valence shell
    b) has firmly bounded electrons
    c) has one electron in its outermost shell
    d) none of the above are correct   _____

27. The rate at which current is delivered is measured in:
    a) amperes   c) volts
    b) ohms   d) watts   _____

28. An ohm is:
    a) the unit used to measure a material's resistance to the flow of
       electric current
    b) the unit used to measure the rate of energy consumption,
       including electric energy
    c) the rate at which current is delivered
    d) the unit used to measure the rate of flow of an electrical current _____

29. An ampere is:
    a) the unit used to measure the rate of flow of an electrical current
    b) the unit used to measure the rate of energy consumption, including
       electric energy
    c) the rate at which current is delivered
    d) the unit used to measure a material's resistance to the flow
       of electric current   _____

30. A watt is:
    a) the unit used to measure the rate of flow of an electrical current
    b) the unit used to measure the rate of energy consumption, including
       electric energy
    c) the rate at which current is delivered
    d) the unit used to measure a material's resistance to the flow
       of electric current   _____

31. The spark created from touching a doorknob is an example of:
    a) static electricity   c) indirect current
    b) direct current   d) alternating current   _____

32. Sinusoidal current is the same as:
    a) static electricity   c) indirect current
    b) direct current   d) alternating current   _____

33. Electrolysis is an example of:
    a) static electricity   c) indirect current
    b) direct current   d) alternating current   _____

34. Galvanic current is an example of:
    a) static electricity   c) indirect current
    b) direct current   d) alternating current   _____

35. High frequency machines use:
    a) static electricity   c) indirect current
    b) direct current   d) alternating current   _____

36. The hertz measures:
    a) the rate of flow of an electrical current
    b) the rate of energy consumption, including electric energy
    c) the rate at which current is delivered
    d) the rate at which the reversal of direction occurs in
       alternating current   _____

37. What type of current is used in US households?
    a) static electricity   c) indirect current
    b) direct current   d) alternating current   _____

38. Which type of current has no polarity?
    a) static electricity   c) alternating current
    b) direct current   d) none of the above
                                      are correct   _____

39. All esthetic machines use:
    a) direct current   c) a and b are correct
    b) alternating current   d) neither a nor b is correct   _____

40. The most important factor when working with electrical devices is:
    a) effectiveness
    b) efficiency
    c) machine usage
    d) safety _____

41. It is advisable to:
    a) use an adapter when you can
    b) modify the plug
    c) overload the circuits
    d) none of the above
       are correct _____

42. Which appliance will most likely use 220 volts?
    a) the high frequency machine
    b) the galvanic machine
    c) the steamer
    d) the dryer _____

Chapter *10*

FIRST IMPRESSIONS – SETUP AND SUPPLIES

1. A thorough tour of the spa should be given to:
   a) first-time callers
   b) only clients who return for a second treatment
   c) clients who have proven themselves to be regulars
   d) only those who ask, because tours are time-consuming

   a

2. Guidelines for first-time callers include:
   a) explaining general protocols for first-time treatments
   b) introducing the client to other members of the team
   c) arriving 15-20 minutes before the treatment
   d) all of the above are correct

   d

3. The 5 R's from the nursing field include all but:
   a) review   c) rewind
   b) reassure   d) record

   c

4. Before a treatment, clients should always remove:
   a) contact lenses   c) socks
   b) bobby pins   d) all of the above are correct

   a

5. The flat sheet on the facial bed is draped:
   a) over the facial bed first   c) over the fitted sheet
   b) over the bed warmer   d) over the blanket

   d

6. A large towel may be used instead of:
   a) the bed warmer   c) a light blanket
   b) the fitted sheet d) the flat sheet

   d

7. What would a sackcloth towel be used for?
   a) wrapping around the clients' feet to keep them warm
   b) hot towel to remove excess product
   c) as a head covering
   d) none of the above are correct

   C

8. Bed warmers should be placed:
   a) under all the bed linens
   b) on top of the client
   c) on top of the fitted sheet
   d) on top of the blanket

   a

9. Noncocoon draping omits the:
   a) bed warmer
   b) fitted sheet
   c) flat sheet
   d) light blanket

   d

10. The main difference in cocoon and noncocoon draping is the:
    a) bed warmer
    b) fitted sheet
    c) flat sheet
    d) light blanket

    d

11. Which is appropriate for using products in the treatment spa?
    a) palette
    b) pumps
    c) squeeze bottles
    d) all of the above are correct

    d

12. A disadvantage of a palette is:
    a) it comes in only one size, regardless of amount of product needed
    b) it is difficult to clean and sanitize
    c) it is not available in plastic, just metal
    d) it is time-consuming

    d

13. Sponges are never:
    a) used on different clients
    b) used to remove eye makeup
    c) dampened before use
    d) left out to dry

    b

14. Sponges should be sanitized by:
    a) dryer
    b) autoclave
    c) chemical solutions
    d) washing machines

    C

15. During the mask treatment waiting period, the esthetician should NOT:
    a) consult with the client on diet and exercise practice
    b) fill in the treatment record chart
    c) plan a home maintenance regimen
    d) retrieve the recommended retail products

    a

16. Advantages of keeping products in the treatment room include:
    a) the products' proximity to the esthetician
    b) appearance
    c) no waste
    d) inventory control

    a

17. A disadvantage of the medical dispensary model is:
    a) less economical method of product usage
    b) theft of product and supplies
    c) disruption to the client
    d) inventory control

    C

18. Microwaves should NOT be used to heat:
    a) solutions   c) hard wax
    b) absorbent cotton   d) hot towels

    d

19. Overheating massage creams in a microwave can cause:
    a) no damage
    b) the product to separate
    c) sparks
    d) increased effectiveness of active ingredients

    b

20. Laundry facilities are best kept:
    a) on the same floor as where the laundry is generated
    b) as far away as possible from the treatment rooms
    c) in the basement
    d) as an outsourced cost

    a

Fornication
Under
Consent of
the King

Chapter *11*

SKIN TYPES AND CONDITIONS

1. Which of the following is NOT a skin type?
   - a) normal
   - b) tertiary skin
   - c) dry/dehydrated skin
   - d) sensitive skin

   B

2. The primary determinant of skin skin types is:
   - a) secretions
   - b) blood type
   - c) lentigenes
   - d) personal preference

   A

3. Skin's moisture retention is determined by:
   - a) t-zones
   - b) telangiectasia
   - c) lipid secretions
   - d) the brand of products used

   C

4. The lipid barrier:
   - a) stays the same through life
   - b) increases with age
   - c) decreases with age
   - d) varies widely from day to day

   C

5. Normal skin:
   - a) requires the least treatment
   - b) is the most common
   - c) appears perfect
   - d) does not age

   C

6. Creams in combination skin systems are:
   - a) higher in oil
   - b) higher in water
   - c) higher in lipids
   - d) lower in water

   B

7. Dehydrated skin:
   - a) is the same as dry skin
   - b) is the same as sensitive skin
   - c) is any type of skin that lacks water
   - d) is any type of skin that lacks oil

   C

8. The treatment for oily skin is to:
   a) dry it
   b) dehydrate it
   c) balance it
   d) moisturize it

   C

9. Dry skin:
   a) lacks oil
   b) lacks water
   c) has intense lipid secretions
   d) is the same as sensitive skin

   A

10. Oily skin:
    a) forms wrinkles easily
    b) responds well to excessive drying treatments
    c) is also known as acne
    d) commonly has clogged follicles

    D

11. Sensitive skin is:
    a) sallow
    b) flaky
    c) pink-to-red
    d) allergic

    C

12. The main goal in treating sensitive skin is to:
    a) exfoliate and cleanse
    b) calm and strengthen the tissue
    c) balance
    d) increase the hydration level

    B

13. Skin conditions:
    a) occur only in oily skin
    b) occur only in dry skin
    c) occur only in sensitive skin
    d) occur in all types of skin

    D

14. Dry skin and dehydrated skin are:
    a) skin types, but not skin conditions
    b) skin conditions, but not skin types
    c) both skin types and skin conditions
    d) the same as sensitive skin

    C

15. Which of the following is an example of hyperpigmentation?
    a) wrinkles
    b) moles
    c) telangiectasia
    d) lentigenes

    D

16. Telangiectasia is the result of:
    a) distended capillaries
    b) hypopigmentation
    c) decreases in the lipid barrier
    d) sun damage

    A

17. The major factor in wrinkle formation is:
    a) excess sebum production
    c) lentigenes
    b) sun exposure
    d) telangiectasia

    B

18. Lymphatic drainage can help in the treatment of:
    a) couperose
    c) wrinkles
    b) moles
    d) puffy eyes

    D

19. Alipidic skin:
    a) is dehydrated
    c) lacks sebum
    b) is oily
    d) none of the above
       are correct

    D

Chapter *12*

HEALTH SCREENING

1. The client's entire health analysis begins with a(n):
   a) health intake form
   b) interactive or conversational analysis
   c) visual analysis
   d) tactile analysis

   A

2. An example of epilation is:
   a) waxing
   b) electrolysis
   c) laser hair removal
   d) all of the above are correct

   D

3. The most important reason for obtaining health information on a written form is:
   a) so that estheticians may prepare for the client's appointment
   b) to periodically check and monitor a client's progress
   c) to avoid liability and harm to the client
   d) to ensure that the client is aware of the procedures involved

   C

4. Photo aging occurs when:
   a) the skin ages due to too much makeup used in photo sessions
   b) the skin ages due to infrared rays used in photo sessions
   c) the skin ages due to sun damage
   d) skin cancer develops due to sun exposure

   C

5. Pregnant women can be quite safe having:
   a) their choice of essential oils during treatments
   b) their choice of body treatments
   c) their choice of facial massage
   d) none of the above are correct

   C

6. Hormonal therapies:
   a) have only negative skin effects
   b) have only positive skin effects
   c) have both positive and negative skin effects
   d) It is not yet known what effect hormonal therapies
      have on the skin.

   C

7. Ortho Tri-Cyclen birth control pills:
   a) can cause acne outbreaks
   b) can be used to treat acne
   c) have the same effects on the skin as other birth control pills
   d) have no effect on the skin

   B

8. Which of these phases can easily cause hyperpigmentation due
   to fluctuating hormones?
   a) I-puberty   c) IV-premenstrual
   b) III-stress   d) V-pregnancy

   D

9. Galvanic, high frequency, and microcurrent treatments are
   contraindicated for:
   a) clients with acne
   b) clients who take birth control pills
   c) clients who are pregnant
   d) clients with asthma

   C

10. Hyperpigmentation has been linked to:
    a) birth control pills   c) a and b are correct
    b) hormone replacement   d) neither a nor b is correct

    C

11. Hormonal therapy patients before or after menopause may
    experience:
    a) less unwanted hair
    b) reduced appearance of wrinkling
    c) softer skin
    d) all of the above are correct

    D

12. Some birth control pills can:
    a) cause breakouts   c) cause hyperpigmentation
    b) clear up hormonal acne   d) all of the above are correct

    D

13. Contact lenses are safe for:
    a) the client having a European facial
    b) 20-minute microdermabrasion treatments
    c) high frequency after extractions
    d) none of the above are correct

    A

14. To ensure safety, contact lenses can be worn only if:
    a) the client is having the routine facial, using no advanced treatments
    b) high frequency is used for a short time
    c) the client insists, and takes responsibility
    d) all of the above are correct

    A

15. In general, the most appropriate treatment for all clients with respect to safety would be:
    a) nonelectric treatment   c) stimulating products
    b) deep tissue massage   d) all of the above are correct

    A

16. Clients using Retin A should NOT have which facial treatment(s)?
    a) sulphur mask and light massage
    b) lymphatic drainage only
    c) waxing only
    d) light massage and waxing

    C

17. A patient who recently had chemotherapy should be especially careful with having:
    a) light massage   c) lymphatic drainage
    b) mud masks   d) all of the above are correct

    C

18. The general rule for electrical treatments is:
    a) When in doubt, ask the client if she has had the treatment before.
    b) When in doubt, only do it if you have done it for clients with similar conditions.
    c) When in doubt, do it.
    d) When in doubt, don't do it.

    D

19. Clients taking antibiotics should NOT receive:
    a) stimulating treatments   c) steam
    b) hydrating treatments   d) extractions

    A

20. Which drug can a patient use safely while receiving a chemical exfoliation?
    a) Prozac   c) Tazorac
    b) Retin A   d) Differin

    A

21. Keratolytic drugs can cause skin to be:
    a) more permeable
    b) more sensitive to pain
    c) a and b are correct
    d) neither a nor b is correct

    C

22. Keratolytic agents are safely used with:
    a) all essential oils
    b) fragranced products
    c) alcohol-based products
    d) none of the above
       are correct

    D

23. Erythmic skin is skin that:
    a) is allergic to the product
    b) hyperpigments with irritants
    c) breaks out with heavy creams, oils, and other rich moisturizers
    d) turns red easily

    D

24. Erythmic skin is an indicator to avoid:
    a) heavy creams, oils, and rich moisturizers
    b) lavender essential oils
    c) lactic-based cleansers
    d) keratolytic agents

    D

25. The drug tretinoin can be found in:
    a) Tazorac
    b) Azelex
    c) Renova
    d) Differin

    C

26. Clients using tretinoin must avoid:
    a) waxing
    b) heat and heat-producing products
    c) fragranced alcohol
    d) all of the above are correct

    D

27. Clients using Accutane need to be even more careful, since Accutane:
    a) is used for infectious diseases
    b) affects the skin of the entire body and stays in the body for long periods
    c) is an antidepressant, and clients may behave unpredictably to treatments
    d) is addictive, and clients using it may need counseling

    B

28. What kind of effect does Accutane have on the body?
    a) keratolytic
    b) severe erythema
    c) blistering
    d) diuretic

    A

29. An example of a systemic drug is:
    a) Accutane
    b) Prednisone
    c) a and b are correct
    d) neither a nor b is correct

    C

30. An example of a topical keratolytic is:
    a) Accutane
    b) Prednisone
    c) Retin A
    d) Benadryl

    C

31. Clients using topical keratolytics on the face can still:
    a) have a disincrustation facial
    b) wax their legs
    c) do a gentle chemical peel
    d) none of the above are correct

    B

32. The best way to determine if someone has AIDS is:
    a) through discreetly asking on the health form
    b) through politely asking privately
    c) assessing the skin yourself for unusual rashes, lesions, etc.
    d) none of the above are correct

    D

33. Hepatitis is a disease that causes:
    a) inflammation of the blood
    b) inflammation of the liver
    c) deterioration of the white blood cells
    d) a lack of blood clotting

    B

34. In a spa, people with active hepatitis should be:
    a) treated if given specific written direction from their doctor
    b) treated by an esthetician with authorization from her doctor
    c) avoided since hepatitis is highly contagious
    d) referred to a dermatologist for professional treatment

    A

35. A chronic disorder is always:
    a) very severe
    b) short-lived
    c) related to the skin
    d) ongoing

    D

36. Which of these is NOT a chronic disorder?
    a) measles
    b) eczema
    c) psoriasis
    d) seborrheic dermatitis

    A

37. What would you recommend with seborrheic dermatitis?
    a) rich and heavy creams
    b) intensive massage
    c) herbal fragranced products
    d) none of the above are correct

    D

38. Lupus patients can safely undergo which treatment without too much caution?
    a) epilation   c) steaming
    b) extraction   d) exfoliation

    C

39. Clients with high blood pressure may have:
    a) redness of the face   c) facial swelling
    b) couperose   d) all of the above are correct

    D

40. Clients who experience edema are:
    a) having colon cleansing   c) having swelling
    b) taking steroids   d) breaking out in hives

    C

41. With proper sanitation, clients with herpes simplex can be treated with:
    a) basic facials   c) a and b are correct
    b) microdermabrasion   d) neither a nor b is correct

    A

42. Who can benefit from taking prophylactic treatments before visiting the spa?
    a) clients with hepatitis   c) clients with herpes simplex
    b) clients with AIDS   d) clients with acne

    C

43. Taking prophylactic drugs 1-2 weeks before an appointment allows the herpes simplex client to:
    a) have alphahydroxy acid peels
    b) have a microdermabrasion facial
    c) a and b are correct
    d) neither a nor b is correct

    C

44. Clients who suffer from sever headaches should avoid:
    a) steam   c) massage
    b) iontophoresis   d) clay based masks

    B

45. Hemophilia is a disease in which:
    a) the liver becomes inflamed
    b) the blood has contracted a rare viral infection
    c) there are not enough white blood cells produced normally
    d) the blood does not clot normally

    D

46. An example of facial surgery that is elective is:
    a) scar revisions after a burn
    b) an eyelid lift to revamp sagging eye muscles
    c) dermabrasion for post cystic acne
    d) all of the above are correct

    B

47. Where does skin cancer rank in terms of prevalence amongst cancer types in the United States?
    a) first   c) third
    b) second   d) last

    A

48. Women who have acne or rosacea tend to also have:
    a) heavy drinking habits   c) stress
    b) lots of spicy foods   d) all of the above are correct

    C

49. Clients that are more likely to have allergies tend to have:
    a) thin, dry, erythmic skin
    b) thick, oily skin, with heavy melanin
    c) aging, sagging skin, with fine lines and wrinkles
    d) none of the above are correct

    A

50. The number one cosmetic allergen is:
    a) fragrance   c) aloe vera
    b) sunscreen chemicals   d) peanut oil

    A

51. What causes flare up and pimples as a result of trying a new product or ingredient?
    a) allergen   c) acnegenic substance
    b) irritant   d) manmade chemicals

    C

52. Clients allergic to aspirin should avoid:
    a) wintergreen   c) filipendula extract
    b) willow bark   d) all of the above are correct

    D

53. Salicylic acid should be avoided on clients allergic to:
    a) peanuts   c) aspirin
    b) chamomile   d) acnegenic substances

    C

54. Patch tests should be performed on what part of the body?
    a) behind the ear or inside the arm
    b) on the palms of the hand or on top of the feet
    c) on any pulse point, as long as the pulse can be felt
    d) on a small area of the face, which is most sensitive

55. How is the client ensured her information is kept confidential?
    a) She chooses a spa with integrity and a good reputation.
    b) Confidentiality is regulated by the Day Spa Association.
    c) The medical disclaimer section of the client form assures this.
    d) There is no assurance of confidentiality with information in spas.

56. What should you do if a client refuses to fill out the health form?
    a) Leave it in her file, and ensure that she fills it out on her next scheduled visit.
    b) Read it through with her, and allow her to answer verbally.
    c) Only allow nonstimulating treatments, such as a basic facial, to be done.
    d) Politely refuse to treat the client to any services.

Chapter *13*

SKIN ANALYSIS

1. The most effective devices for skin analysis include all except:
   a) eyes
   b) loupe
   c) sense of smell
   d) hands

   C

2. Conditions of using a Wood's Lamp include:
   a) having a well lit room
   b) having exposure to natural sunlight
   c) holding the skin firmly
   d) having a dark room

   d

3. A loupe is the same as a:
   a) mag light
   b) ultraviolet light
   c) infrared lamp
   d) microscope

   a

4. Which skin condition is visible with the Wood's lamp?
   a) hypopigmentation
   b) lint
   c) bacteria
   d) all of the above are correct

   C

5. A fungus on the skin will show on the Wood's Lamp as:
   a) white specks
   b) pinkish to orangish dots
   c) bright or neon yellow
   d) A fungus will not show up as a skin condition under the Wood's Lamp.

   C

6. Which is NOT used by the esthetician to analyze the skin?
   a) hands
   b) loupe
   c) microscope
   d) skin scanner

   C

7. When does skin analysis begin for the esthetician?
   a) when the client arrives, still in makeup
   b) when the cleansing begins
   c) when the makeup is removed
   d) when the magnifying lamp is turned on and you can see
      through the loupe

   a

8. When should skin analysis end?
   a) when the mag light is turned off and extractions begin
   b) before you begin the relaxing massage
   c) just before putting on day cream and sunscreen
   d) at the client's departure

   d

9. What can be part of a visual checklist for men?
   a) ingrown hairs
   b) any irritation on the skin or neck
   c) thick or pinkish skin on a receding hairline
   d) all of the above are correct

   d

10. Which of these is useful in assessing a female client before the
    treatment?
    a) hairstyle
    b) clothing
    c) overall gestures and atmosphere
    d) all of the above are correct

    d

11. What is the main difference between a quick cleanse and a full
    cleanse?
    a) they are the same, except the quick cleanse does faster rotations,
       and the full cleanse does slower
    b) the full cleanse repeats the steps of the quick cleanse twice to
       remove any residue
    c) they are the same except the quick cleanse does not use a
       freshener after makeup removal, and the full cleanse does
    d) none of the above are correct

    c

12. Charting, in the health care industry, means:
    a) scheduling appointments in consecutive time gaps, such as weekly
       or fortnightly
    b) prioritizing client appointments, with the most urgent being
       booked first
    c) recording information regarding a client
    d) portraying client progress in graphic forms

    c

13. Who is usually responsible for charting in a spa?
    a) spa director
    b) esthetician
    c) front desk personnel
    d) spa attendant

    b

14. Which of these is initially in a client's chart?
    a) health forms
    b) treatment forms
    c) skin analysis forms
    d) all of the above are correct

    d

15. Which of these is NOT obtained from a client's chart?
    a) complete freedom from litigation
    b) complete details on a client's skin type and conditions
    c) home skin care regimen
    d) legal documentation on a client

    a

16. Noticeable telangiectasia will be documented under which sub-section of the skin analysis form?
    a) peripheral vascular system and its disorders
    b) lipid systems and their disorders
    c) hydric system and its disorders
    d) excrescences

    a

17. A pregnancy mask is known as:
    a) vitiligo
    b) senile lentigo
    c) nevus epidermal
    d) chloasma

    d

18. Vitiligo is a:
    a) nonpigmented patch
    b) liver spot
    c) mole
    d) birth mark

    a

19. Which of these would fall under the peripheral vascular system and its disorders?
    a) cyanosis
    b) hyperkeratinization
    c) seborrhea
    d) all of the above are correct

    a

20. Which of these is NOT a pigmentation disorder?
    a) vitiligo
    b) senile lentigo
    c) nevus epidermal
    d) chloasma

    c

21. Which of these is a red, round swelling, a disorder of the peripheral vascular system?
    a) erythema
    b) erythrosis
    c) angioma
    d) ephelides

    c

22. Crusty inflammation on the skin is described as:
    a) hyperkeratinization   c) eczema
    b) furfur   d) ichthyosis   *C*

23. Nodules and papules belong to the category of:
    a) complexion and pigment disorders
    b) the hydric system and its disorders
    c) the peripheral vascular system and its disorders
    d) the lipid system and its disorders   *d*

24. If seborrhea were noticed on a client, what category would this
    be in?
    a) the lipid system and its disorders
    b) the hydric system and its disorders
    c) the peripheral vascular system and its disorders
    d) keratinization   *a*

25. The grain of the skin can be described as:
    a) the moisture level of the skin   c) the tan and phototypes
    b) the thickness of the skin   d) the size of the pore   *d*

26. Wrinkles are a disorder of the:
    a) hydric system   c) peripheral vascular system
    b) lipid system   d) none of the above
                                        are correct   *a*

27. Hypertrichosis is a disorder of:
    a) the lipid system   c) skin sensitivity
    b) the hydric system   d) the hair system   *d*

28. When assessing skin hydration, you will be looking for:
    a) furrows   c) pruritus
    b) moles   d) acne   *a*

29. When assessing skin keratinization, you will be looking for:
    a) furfur   c) senile lentigo
    b) pruritis   d) chloasma   *a*

30. In assessing for lipid disorders, you'll be looking for:
    a) erythrosis   c) asphyxiation
    b) angioma   d) ephelis   *C*

31. Vascular and follicular dilation is better known as:
    a) eryhtrosis
    b) couperose
    c) cyanosis
    d) angioma

    b

32. Folliculitis and furuncles are both caused by:
    a) a fungus
    b) bacteria
    c) a virus
    d) keratinization

    b

33. A common boil is also termed:
    a) vitiligo
    b) phlycena
    c) ephelides
    d) furuncle

    d

34. Which of these is a pigmentation disorder?
    a) vitiligo
    b) ephelides
    c) chloasma
    d) all of the above are correct

    d

35. Which of the following describes complexion?
    a) amber
    b) bluish
    c) yellow-green
    d) creamy

    a

Chapter 14

ANATOMY OF A FACIAL

1. The first phase of the facial is always:
   a) light cleansing
   b) massage
   c) skin analysis using the magnifying lamp
   d) mask application

   A

2. The last phase of the facial is always:
   a) massage
   b) applying a mask
   c) applying moisturizer and sunblock
   d) applying toner and freshener

   C

3. Facials can benefit the skin by:
   a) increasing blood and lymph circulation
   b) prevention against premature aging of the skin
   c) relaxation
   d) all of the above are correct

   D

4. Which of these readjusts the skin's pH level?
   a) cleanser   c) day cream
   b) freshener   d) steam

   B

5. Which of these is most effective in drawing out impurities while tightening and toning the skin?
   a) steam   c) foaming cleanser
   b) mask   d) all of the above are correct

   B

6. Which of these is NOT alkaline in nature?
   a) makeup remover   c) a and b are correct
   b) foaming cleanser d) neither a nor b is correct

   B

7. A standard facial is normally divided into how many steps?

   a) 3   c) 7

   b) 5   d) 9   C

8. A necessary step that should be taken to prepare for the client is:

   a) to prepare the facial chair with fresh linens and covering

   b) to fill the steamer with boiling water and preheat it with ozone off

   c) to place the glass electrode into the hand device of the high frequency machine beforehand

   d) all of the above are correct   D

9. How do you correctly remove mascara from a client's eyelashes?

   a) It is always better to ask the client politely to remove it before the treatment.

   b) With the client's eyes closed, place the lashes between swabs and swipe down and away from eye and lash.

   c) With the client's eyes open, place the lashes between swabs and swipe down and away from eye and lash.

   d) With the client's eyes closed, use a cotton pad and rub gently back and forth.   B

10. The magnifying light should be positioned between:

    a) 2-4 inches away from the client

    b) 4-6 inches away from the client

    c) 6-12 inches away from the client

    d) 12-15 inches away from the client   C

11. In a 50-minute facial, an entire analysis, including using the magnifying light, touching, Wood's lamp, and conversing with the client, should take:

    a) less than 1 minute   c) 5-7 minutes

    b) 3-5 minutes   d) 7-10 minutes   C

12. When using the brush machine, begin at:

    a) the forehead and work downward

    b) the sides of the face and move inward

    c) the neck and work up the face

    d) the forehead and go down the T-zone area first   C

13. Before turning on the galvanic machine, place the electrode:

    a) in the center of the forehead   c) in the chin area

    b) in the nose area   d) on one of the eyelids   A

14. In a standard 50-minute facial, extractions should last:
    a) 5 minutes
    b) 10 minutes
    c) 15 minutes
    d) as long as it takes to clean the face thoroughly of comedones *A*

15. A facial massage:
    a) relaxes the client
    b) stimulates cell turnover
    c) helps to infuse any ampoule concentrate
    d) all of the above are correct *D*

16. Thermal masks:
    a) are stored in heated areas to preserve their healing properties
    b) are heated prior to use to release their healing properties
    c) are applied with a hot towel placed on top of them to heat them up
    d) become warm when applied to the skin, and cool as they harden *D*

17. Where should you begin applying the mask?
    a) the forehead and work downward
    b) the sides of the face and move inward
    c) the neck and work up the face
    d) the forehead and go down the T-zone area first *C*

18. Which of these does a facial massage NOT do?
    a) help muscle tone
    b) activate sluggish skin
    c) increase sebum production
    d) help cleanse skin of impurities *C*

19. Tapotement is often referred to as:
    a) percussion   c) tapping *A*
    b) friction   d) none of the above are correct

20. A "classical" massage is also known as:
    a) acupressure   c) Swedish *C*
    b) shiatsu   d) lymph drainage

21. Which massage technique uses gentle pressure to remove waste materials from the body? *D*
    a) acupressure   c) reflexology
    b) shiatsu   d) lymph drainage

22. Which massage form is focused only on the hands and feet?
    a) acupressure   c) reflexology
    b) shiatsu   d) lymphatic drainage

    C

23. A facial is performed for approximately:
    a) 5–10 minutes   c) 15–20 minutes
    b) 10–15 minutes   d) 20–25 minutes

    B

24. The massage which combines the stretching of the limbs with pressure on points is called:
    a) acupressure   c) reflexology
    b) shiatsu   d) lymphatic drainage

    B

25. The massage most appropriate for oily skin is:
    a) acupressure   c) the Dr. Jacquet method
    b) lymphatic drainage   d) aromatherapy

    C

26. Classical massage movements do NOT include:
    a) friction   c) vibration
    b) reflexology   d) tapotement

    B

27. The massage movement used by most estheticians to open and close the facial massage period is:
    a) effleurage   c) tapotement
    b) friction   d) petrissage

    A

28. Chucking, rolling, and wringing are variations of:
    a) effleurage   c) vibration
    b) tapotement   d) friction

    D

29. Which movement is considered most important to the esthetician?
    a) effleurage   c) vibration
    b) tapotement   d) friction

    A

30. Which movement should be used sparingly in facial massage, since it is the most stimulating movement?
    a) petrissage   c) vibration
    b) tapotement   d) friction

    B

31. Which movement is used mainly to stimulate sebum production?
    a) petrissage   c) vibration
    b) tapotement   d) friction

    A

32. The piano movement is described as:
    a) light digital tapping on the face
    b) pressure points on the face
    c) slow, rhythmic movements on the face
    d) a shaking movement done lightly, emanating from the shoulders

    A

33. Which movement is suitable for the scalp, arms, and hands?
    a) petrissage   c) vibration
    b) tapotement   d) friction

    D

34. A friction movement in which the esthetician's hands are placed
    a little distance apart on both sides, moving the flesh in opposite
    directions, is:
    a) rolling   c) chucking
    b) wringing   d) slapping

    B

35. Chucking, rolling, and wringing are employed mainly to massage the:
    a) scalp and neck area   c) back and thighs
    b) muscles of the abdomen d) arms and legs

    D

36. What part of the body is used to employ the hacking movement
    on a client?
    a) wrists and outer edges of the hands
    b) wrists and inner edges of the hands
    c) wrists and palms of the hand
    d) none of the above are correct

    A

37. How many basic facial types are there to correspond to the basic
    skin types?
    a) 3   c) 5
    b) 4   d) 7

    A

38. Which of the following skin types would NOT have Phase IV
    (treat and correct) of the facial steps?
    a) normal skin   c) normal/combination
    b) dry/dehydrated skin   d) sensitive skin

    A

39. Which skin type needs dead cells exfoliated, lost moisture replenished, and the restoring (lubricating) of the skin's moisture barrier?
    a) normal skin
    b) normal/combination
    c) dry/dehydrated skin
    d) none of the above are correct

    C

40. The high frequency machine is used on:
    a) all skin types
    b) only oily skins and combination skins
    c) normal/combination and dry/dehydrated skins
    d) dry/dehydrated skins only

    C

41. Massage dates back about:
    a) 100 years
    b) 500 years
    c) 1,000 years
    d) 3,000 years

    D

42. Minifacials always include:
    a) masking
    b) massage
    c) a and b are correct
    d) neither a nor b is correct

    A

43. Performing all the steps of the minifacial should take:
    a) 15 minutes
    b) 20 minutes
    c) 25 minutes
    d) 30 minutes

    C

44. How long do you leave the mask on for a minifacial?
    a) You do NOT apply a mask in a minifacial.
    b) 5 minutes
    c) 10 minutes
    d) 15 minutes

    B

45. Which step is omitted in a minifacial?
    a) applying freshener after the mask
    b) filling out the complete home care chart
    c) follow-up courtesy call after 1-2 days
    d) none of the above are correct

    D

46. Which of these is included in a minifacial?
    a) skin analysis with a Wood's lamp
    b) 5 minutes of pressure point massage
    c) extractions
    d) recommending home care retail and filling out home care chart

    D

47. The function of a toner is to:
     a) prevent dehydration of the skin
     b) protect the skin against sunlight
     c) camouflage the complexion
     d) remove oil from the skin after cleansing

48. Qualities of skin cleanser include:
     a) cleanse the skin effectively, without causing irritation
     b) remove all traces of makeup and grease
     c) easy to remove from the skin
     d) all of the above are correct

Chapter **15**

MEN'S FACIAL

1. Male clients can be beneficial to the spa because they are:
   a) more willing to follow suggestions
   b) loyal customers
   c) happy for basic, consistent routines
   d) all of the above are correct

   D

2. Men now comprise about:
   a) 10% of the market
   b) 15-20% of the market
   c) 25-30% of the market
   d) 40% of the market

   B

3. Which of these would a man generally prefer?
   a) a lavender-scented cleanser
   b) creams that leave a dewy, shiny look
   c) two-in-one cleanser and toner
   d) none of the above are correct

   C

4. Which is true about men's taste, generally?
   a) They prefer jars to tubes.
   b) They like foamy cleansers.
   c) a and b are correct
   d) neither a nor b is correct

   B

5. The two top retail items to sell a man initially would be:
   a) cleanser and toner
   b) cleanser and moisturizer
   c) cleanser and mask
   d) moisturizer and mask

   B

6. Items that should be added later to his home regimen include:
   a) cleanser and mask
   b) moisturizer and mask
   c) sunscreen and mask
   d) sunscreen and moisturizer

   C

7. Men who have experienced irritation from shaving are
   advised to:
   a) dry shave instead
   b) wax their facial hair
   c) grow their facial hair
   d) shave in the same direction as the hair growth   *D*

8. Most men will NOT enjoy:
   a) the steamer on their face
   b) the brush machine to exfoliate
   c) cleansing with warm cotton pads
   d) all of the above are correct   *C*

9. Men with sensitive skin who have just shaved should be
   cautious with:
   a) exfoliating chemicals   c) microdermabrasion
   b) alpha hydroxy acids   d) all of the above are correct   *D*

10. Most massage movements on the beard area should be:
    a) circular and rhythmic
    b) upward against gravity
    c) downward, in the direction of the hair growth
    d) all of the above are correct   *C*

11. Men can be susceptible to folliculitis if they:
    a) have a coarse or wiry beard
    b) shave in the direction of the hair growth
    c) a and b are correct
    d) neither a nor b is correct   *A*

12. Folliculitis should be treated by:
    a) alleviating the irritation
    b) drying up and disinfecting the area
    c) desensitizing the area
    d) all of the above are correct   *D*

13. Men are least likely to wax:
    a) brows   c) mustache
    b) nape of the neck   d) back   *C*

14. Appealing scents for hot towels for the male client include:
    a) citrus   c) a and b are correct
    b) menthol   d) neither a nor b is correct

    C

15. Masks are kept on for how long for male clients?
    a) 5-7 minutes   c) 10-15 minutes
    b) 7-10 minutes   d) 15-20 minutes

    B

Chapter 16

POSTCONSULTATION AND HOME CARE

1. About what percentage of sales is generated from retail in a successful spa?
   a) 17%
   b) 25%
   c) 33%
   d) 40%

   D

2. The best way to overcome your fear of selling is by:
   a) realizing that everyone else is a salesman too, so you need to get a piece of the pie
   b) rehearsing your lines and taking deep breaths
   c) doing it on the phone in the follow-up call
   d) realizing that you are serving customers

   D

3. When selling a product effectively:
   a) explain the features of the product, such as its ingredients, shelf life, etc.
   b) educate clients on its personal benefits
   c) a and b are correct
   d) neither a nor b is correct

   B

4. Postconsultation and home care is the part of the facial that:
   a) will help you make the most money
   b) shows clients that you care about their skin
   c) clients appreciate the least
   d) don't impact skin health

   B

5. How often, if ever, should a home care chart be written up?
   a) it does not need to be changed but is always effective
   b) no more than once a year
   c) at least two to four times a year for seasonal changes in routine
   d) whenever the client returns, she should be reexamined and a new chart should be done

   C

6. Which is NOT a step in postconsultation?
   a) developing a long-term program
   b) recommending a home care regimen
   c) using a Wood's lamp
   d) making a follow-up phone call

   C

7. The five-minute close allows the esthetician to:
   a) address a client's concerns that were written on the health form
   b) make suggestions about optional treatments and products
   c) discuss what the client would like to accomplish for the future
   d) all of the above are correct

   D

8. The key to a successful skin care program is:
   a) to see the client for more than one treatment
   b) for the client to use the most expensive products
   c) incorporating the spa's products into the client's regime
   d) good record-keeping

   A

9. The purpose of the postconsultation is to:
   a) show clients you are a true professional who cares about them
   b) take the mystery out of confusing product selection and treatments
   c) a and b are correct
   d) to sell as many products as possible

   C

10. Ideally, the home care guide should include:
    a) how and when to use daily products
    b) the amount of product to use
    c) your contact info
    d) all of the above are correct

    D

11. What should you NEVER do when a client is dedicated to using a brand you do not endorse or know anything about?
    a) learn more about those products
    b) suggest she throw those products out
    c) recommend some corrective products from your line
    d) suggest she replace them with products from your line when she has used all of hers

    B

12. The goal of the closing consultation is to:
    a) sell your product line
    b) show the client how professional you are
    c) show the client how knowledgeable you are
    d) provide information in a straightforward and user-friendly manner

    D

13. How long should the esthetician wait before making a follow up
    call?
    a) 1–2 hours   c) 1–2 weeks
    b) 1–2 days   d) 1–2 months

    B

14. Reasons for making a follow-up call include:
    a) to prevent major problems from happening
    b) to build trust and confidence
    c) a and b are correct
    d) a follow-up call is only necessary in an emergency

    C

15. An important tool in the postconsultation phase of a facial is a:
    a) Wood's lamp   c) health history form
    b) home care guide   d) mag light

    B

16. Which of the following are characteristics of an effective home
    care guide?
    a) attractive presentation
    b) fill-in-the-blank format
    c) a copy for the client's file at the spa
    d) all of the above are correct

    D

17. Clients who don't purchase products or can't be bothered with a
    skin care routine:
    a) are lazy
    b) usually don't understand the values and uses of products
    c) aren't interested
    d) have excellent skin

    B

18. The esthetician should NOT use the home care guide to:
    a) mark the most important products for clients to purchase immediately
    b) recommend your product line in large print
    c) de-emphasize the client's own products with small print
    d) cross out all the client's own products

    D

19. The home care guide should be updated to accommodate
    changes in:
    a) technology   c) lifestyle
    b) age and health   d) all of the above are correct

    D

Chapter 17

DISORDERS AND DISEASES

1. An example of an objective symptom is:
   a) edema
   b) pruritus
   c) burning
   d) all of the above are correct

   a

2. Atopic dermatitis:
   a) has only topical inflammation
   b) is an advanced form of dermatitis
   c) runs in the family
   d) involves severe itching

   c

3. The medical term for itching is:
   a) contact dermatitis
   b) keratosis
   c) psoriasis
   d) pruritus

   d

4. Any form of lesion caused by bleeding is called a:
   a) purpura
   b) hematoma
   c) ecchymoses
   d) none of the above
      are correct

   a

5. Malignant lesions:
   a) are cancerous lesions
   b) are nonpigmented
   c) are contagious
   d) are caused by bleeding

   a

6. Which is NOT a type of lesion?
   a) primary
   b) secondary
   c) tertiary
   d) vascular

   c

7. Scales, crusts, and keloids are examples of:
   a) primary lesions
   b) secondary lesions
   c) malignant lesions
   d) vascular

   b

8. Cherry angioma and telangiectasia fall under the category of:
   a) primary lesions
   b) secondary lesions
   c) vascular lesions
   d) none of the above are correct

   c

9. Terms used to describe lesion shapes include all except:
   a) linear
   b) annular
   c) geographic
   d) historical

   d

10. What does a serpiginous lesion look like?
    a) a target
    b) round
    c) the sun
    d) a snake

    d

11. Which of these statements are (is) true?
    a) a macule is any sort of flat lesion
    b) milia are an example of macules
    c) a and b are correct
    d) neither a nor b is correct

    a

12. The singular form of comedones, or blackheads, is:
    a) comedone
    b) comeda
    c) comedo
    d) comedia

    c

13. The technical term for whiteheads is:
    a) comedones
    b) macules
    c) papules
    d) milia

    d

14. Milia can appear as a result of:
    a) dermabrasion
    b) chemical peels
    c) laser resurfacing
    d) all of the above are correct

    d

15. Acne is an example of:
    a) milia
    b) macules
    c) papules
    d) nodules

    c

16. Nodules can be brought on by:
    a) scar tissue
    b) fatty deposits
    c) a and b are correct
    d) neither a nor b is correct

    c

17. Edematous lesions:
    a) are filled with pus
    b) are filled with liquid
    c) are filled with sebum
    d) are flat

    b

18. A keloid is:
    a) hypertrophic by nature
    b) hereditary, especially prevalent in black and Asian skin
    c) a and b are correct
    d) neither a nor b is correct

    C

19. A port wine stain is a good example of:
    a) bullae
    b) pigmented nevus
    c) vascular nevus
    d) telangiectasia

    C

20. Skin tags, small extensions of skin that hang or flap, can be removed by:
    a) cryosurgery
    b) clipping with surgical scissors
    c) treatment with an electric needle
    d) all of the above are correct

    d

21. Which of these is an inflammatory disorder characterized by erythema and flaking in oilier areas?
    a) seborrhea
    b) seborrheic dermatitis
    c) keratosis pilaris
    d) rosacea

    b

22. Seborrheic dermatitis:
    a) is more prevalent in women than in men
    b) can be treated with the same medication as dandruff
    c) is less likely to develop as you age
    d) is more prevalent in men than in women

    b

23. Rosacea is most common in which skin types, according to the Fitzpatrick Scale?
    a) types I-III
    b) types III-VI
    c) any skin type
    d) type III only

    a

hypertrophic- overgrowth

24. Which of these is true for rosacea?
    a) It occurs in men and women with the same frequency.
    b) Lucas sprays should be avoided when doing facials on rosacea skin.
    c) Anti-yeast medication is commonly used to treat rosacea.
    d) Steamers and hot towels should be used generously on skin with rosacea.

    c

25. Which of these terms describes small clusters of papules around the mouth?
    a) rosacea   c) urticaria
    b) seborrheic dermatitis   d) perioral dermatitis

    d

26. Which of the following statements is true for perioral dermatitis?
    a) It occurs almost exclusively in men.
    b) It can be treated with AHAs.
    c) It is contagious.
    d) none of the above are correct

    d

27. Which of these disorders is contagious?
    a) contact dermatitis   c) perioral dermatitis
    b) irritant contact dermatitis   d) herpes simplex

    d

28. Poison ivy is a good example of:
    a) allergic contact dermatitis   c) perioral dermatitis
    b) irritant contact dermatitis   d) none of the above
                                           are correct

    a

29. The number-one cause of allergic reactions to products is from:
    a) fragrances   c) hives
    b) preservatives   d) essential oils

    a

30. Estheticians may see irritant contact dermatitis in clients who are prone to:
    a) using excess essential oils   c) overuse of acne medication
    b) nasal allergies   d) all of the above are correct

    c

31. Which is true for atopic dermatitis?
    a) It is genetic by nature.
    b) It is worse in summer months.
    c) It is most common in adults on the face and décolleté area.
    d) It is a form of acne.

    a

32. Treatments for atopic dermatitis include:
    a) a one week course of antibiotics
    b) anti-yeast medication
    c) relieving the skin with moisturizers based on essential oils
    d) using corticosteroids *(cortizone cream)*

    d

33. Psoriasis is most prevalent in:
    a) those with autoimmune diseases
    b) those with the hereditary gene
    c) a and b are correct
    d) neither a nor b is correct

    c

34. Atopic dermatitis and psoriasis both:
    a) are hereditary disorders of the skin
    b) affect the legs, elbows, and knees
    c) can be treated with topical corticosteroids
    d) all of the above are correct

    d

35. Which skin condition can you recognize by a pattern of a Christmas tree on the skin?
    a) secondary syphilis   c) a and b are correct
    b) pityriasis rosea   d) neither a nor b are correct

    c

36. Which of these is caused by a virus?
    a) warts   c) keloids
    b) tinea   d) acne

    a

37. Which of these is caused by bacteria?
    a) chicken pox   c) pinkeye
    b) athlete's foot   d) cold sores

    c

38. Cold sores are:
    a) caused by a fungus, called herpes simplex
    b) hereditary by nature
    c) caused by a virus
    d) an allergic reaction

    c

39. Which of these is true for athlete's foot?
    a) It can be avoided by wearing slip-ons and slides in wet areas.
    b) It can be treated with antibiotic creams.
    c) It normally develops at the heel of the foot.
    d) It develops in children only.

    a

40. The white splotches of hypopigmentation on the body is due to the yeast called:
    a) tinea pedis
    b) tinea versicolor
    c) tinea corporis
    d) tinea manis

    _b_

41. Herpes zoster is the virus that causes:
    a) shingles
    b) cold sores
    c) warts
    d) perioral dermatitis

    _a_

42. The skin condition known as cellulitis is:
    a) fatal in severe cases
    b) caused by a virus infection
    c) appears as spongy, "orange peel" skin
    d) present in the thighs only

    _a_

43. Which of these helps prevent folliculitis?
    a) using electric razors
    b) cleansing the skin with salicylic acid based preparations
    c) shaving in the same direction as hair growth
    d) all of the above are correct

    _d_

44. An example of reversible hypopigmentation is:
    a) albinism
    b) vitiligo
    c) tinea versicolor
    d) ephelides

    _c_

45. Age spots are also known as:
    a) mottling
    b) solar lentigines
    c) melasma
    d) PIH

    _b_

46. Estheticians must be especially careful of PIH in skin type(s):
    a) I of the Fitzpatrick scale
    b) II and III of the Fitzpatrick scale
    c) IV, V, and VI of the Fitzpatrick scale
    d) VI of the Fitzpatrick scale

    _c_

47. The only drug currently approved by the FDA to treat hyperpigmentation is:
    a) melanin
    b) kojic acid
    c) licorice extract
    d) hydroquinone

    _d_

48. Which treatment can be used by estheticians to aid in hyperpigmentation disorders?
    a) alpha hydroxy acids
    b) benzoyl peroxide
    c) corticosteroids
    d) antibiotic creams

    a

49. I. Having a depressed immune system is the same as being immunocompromised.
    II. Having a depressed immune system is the same as being immunosuppressed.
    a) I and II are both correct
    b) I is correct, II is incorrect
    c) I is incorrect, II is correct
    d) I and II are both incorrect

    a

50. Systemic lupus erythematosus (SLE) causes a red rash on the face that looks like a:
    a) port wine stain
    b) Christmas tree
    c) ringworm
    d) butterfly

    d

51. Facts about lupus include:
    a) It is improved by sun exposure.
    b) Both types (SLE and DLE) are more prevalent in men.
    c) Discoid lupus, or lupus of the skin, can be treated with malaria drugs.
    d) Systemic lupus erythematosus (SLE) can be treated with antibiotics.

    C

52. The most important treatment to help a lupus patient is to:
    a) treat the patient sensitively
    b) administer gentle hydrating masks
    c) restore the pH balance of the skin
    d) choose an appropriate sunscreen

    d

Chapter *18*

PHARMACOLOGY

1. Pharmacology is defined as:
   a) the study of medicinal drugs, how they work, and how they are prepared
   b) the study of skin disorders, their symptoms, their causes, and drugs to remedy them
   c) the study of prescription drugs, their uses, and their contraindications
   d) the study of the functions of the human body

   A

2. Which of these is NOT an example of OTC drugs sold by estheticians?
   a) sunscreen
   b) acne drugs
   c) lightening products
   d) retin-A gel

   D

3. Zinc oxide and titanium oxide:
   a) are examples of chemical sunscreens
   b) absorb and neutralize UV rays
   c) block a large part of UVA rays
   d) are both used in makeup products

   C

4. Particulate sunscreens:
   a) are not broad-spectrum sunscreens
   b) are made from earth pigments
   c) are examples of chemical sunscreens
   d) absorb and neutralize UVB rays

   B

5. An advantage of an absorbing sunscreen over a reflecting sunscreen is:
   a) it is less irritating to the skin
   b) it absorbs heat while absorbing the rays
   c) it cannot be seen on the skin
   d) it blocks a large part of UVA rays

   C

6. People with combination and oily skin should use sunscreens based in:
   a) a cream
   b) an oil
   c) a noncomedogenic fluid
   d) any of the bases, as long as the SPF is high enough

   C

7. Water-resistant sunscreen has to be effective after being submerged in water for how long?
   a) 30 minutes   c) 120 minutes
   b) 80 minutes   d) 180 minutes

   B

8. When listing ingredients in an OTC drug:
   a) the most expensive ingredients must be placed first
   b) the ingredients must be listed alphabetically
   c) the active ingredients are listed first, with non-drug ingredients after
   d) ingredients are listed in any order that the manufacturer finds effective

   C

9. Which of these ingredients is NOT OTC approved for acne treatment?
   a) sulphur   c) tretinoin
   b) salicylic acid   d) benzoyl peroxide

   C

10. Masks for acne are normally always:
    a) oil-based   c) mud-based
    b) water-based   d) clay-based

    D

11. Estheticians can sell OTC hydroquinone at what strength?
    a) 2%   c) 8%
    b) 4%   d) up to 0.5%

    A

12. Physicians can prescribe which drug for hyperpigmentation?
    a) Solaquin   c) Melanex
    b) Lustra   d) all of the above are correct

    D

13. Corticosteroids are defined as:
    a) tretinoins used to treat inflammatory and cystic acne
    b) OTC drugs that are approved for lightening the skin
    c) hormones that help to relieve inflammation
    d) hormones used to regulate the production of melanin

    C

14. The term "itch and redness relieving drugs" refers to:
    a) triple antibiotic ointments   c) hydrocortisone creams
    b) hydrating creams   d) aloe vera gel

    C

15. Hydrocortisones may be:
    a) used for up to a month at a time, on a daily basis
    b) applied to the eyes
    c) bought at 10% over the counter
    d) bought at up to 1% over the counter

    D

16. If overused, hydrocortisones can:
    a) cause breakouts and aggravate flares
    b) be stored in the body, where it is toxic
    c) cause the skin to thin, resulting in long-range problems
    d) clog the pores

    C

17. Which of these disorders is NOT treated with prescription corti-
    sone products?
    a) poison ivy   c) seborrheic dermatitis
    b) alopecia   d) eczema

    B

18. Which of these prescription steroids is appropriate for use on the
    face?
    a) Temovate   c) Diprolene
    b) Aclovate   d) Psorcon

    B

19. Clients who tell you they use prednisone:
    a) suffer from a severe disease
    b) are using a topical steroid cream
    c) suffer from lupus or other chronic conditions
    d) have severe acne

    C

20. Estheticians who are treating clients using prednisone:
    a) can give the same treatment as for any other client
    b) should not give any stimulating treatments
    c) should treat for acne skin
    d) should not give any treatments; the client should
       see a dermatologist

    B

21. Antihistamines can be used to treat:
    a) urticaria (hives)   c) insect bites
    b) itching   d) all of the above are correct

    D

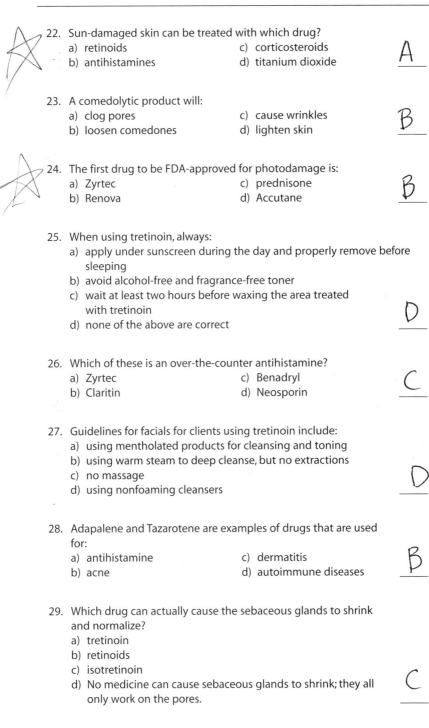

22. Sun-damaged skin can be treated with which drug?
    a) retinoids
    c) corticosteroids
    b) antihistamines
    d) titanium dioxide

    A

23. A comedolytic product will:
    a) clog pores
    c) cause wrinkles
    b) loosen comedones
    d) lighten skin

    B

24. The first drug to be FDA-approved for photodamage is:
    a) Zyrtec
    c) prednisone
    b) Renova
    d) Accutane

    B

25. When using tretinoin, always:
    a) apply under sunscreen during the day and properly remove before sleeping
    b) avoid alcohol-free and fragrance-free toner
    c) wait at least two hours before waxing the area treated with tretinoin
    d) none of the above are correct

    D

26. Which of these is an over-the-counter antihistamine?
    a) Zyrtec
    c) Benadryl
    b) Claritin
    d) Neosporin

    C

27. Guidelines for facials for clients using tretinoin include:
    a) using mentholated products for cleansing and toning
    b) using warm steam to deep cleanse, but no extractions
    c) no massage
    d) using nonfoaming cleansers

    D

28. Adapalene and Tazarotene are examples of drugs that are used for:
    a) antihistamine
    c) dermatitis
    b) acne
    d) autoimmune diseases

    B

29. Which drug can actually cause the sebaceous glands to shrink and normalize?
    a) tretinoin
    b) retinoids
    c) isotretinoin
    d) No medicine can cause sebaceous glands to shrink; they all only work on the pores.

    C

30. Which of these drugs will be least irritating to the skin, according to its active ingredients?
    a) retin-A
    b) Renova
    c) retinol
    d) retinyl palmitate

    D

31. Side effects of Accutane include:
    a) birth defects in children of women taking it
    b) increasing fats in the blood
    c) developing bone and tendon calcification
    d) all of the above are correct

    D

32. Clients using Accutane can safely continue using:
    a) keratolytic products
    b) retinol
    c) soft wax on the legs only
    d) gel hydrating masks

    D

33. Which ingredient is soothing for Accutane users?
    a) azulene
    b) green tea extract
    c) matricaria
    d) all of the above are correct

    D

34. Rosacea can be treated with a prescription:
    a) antiyeast and antihistamine medication
    b) antibiotic only
    c) antibiotics and antiyeast medication
    d) antibiotics and hydrocortisone

    C

35. Metrogel, Metrolotion, and Metrocream all fight rosacea by:
    a) drying up the excess sebum that causes breakouts
    b) reducing redness through filtering out damaging rays
    c) controlling the inflammation and helping to prevent flares
    d) moisturizing the dry areas and preventing flaking

    C

36. Which of these is true for antibiotics?
    a) They help to reduce inflammation.
    b) Topical antibiotics are always prescription drugs.
    c) Bacteria cannot become resistant to antibiotics.
    d) They treat reactions such as hives.

    A

37. Which of these is caused by a virus?
    a) impetigo
    b) cold sores
    c) furuncles
    d) cellulitis

    B

38. Clients using the drug Zovirax can be using it to treat:
    a) cold sores
    c) chicken pox
    b) genital herpes
    d) all of the above are correct

    D

39. When using keratolytic drugs:
    a) avoid alpha hydroxy acids
    b) soothe with essential oils
    c) apply antibacterial toners such as isopropyl alcohol
    d) remove hair with hard wax only

    A

40. Vitamin A is highly present in:
    a) wheat germ oil
    c) AHAs
    b) tretinoin
    d) alpha tocopherol

    B

Chapter 19

PRODUCT CHEMISTRY

1. Chemistry is the study of:
   a) the composition of substances and their effects on one another
   b) the properties of rays and energy
   c) the science of life
   d) living matter

   a

2. One myth in the cosmetics world is that:
   a) all chemicals are bad for the skin
   b) natural ingredients do not contain chemicals
   c) a and b are myths
   d) neither a nor b are myths

   c

3. Applied chemistry is:
   a) the search for practical uses for the knowledge of chemistry
   b) the study of chemical reactions
   c) done only by biochemists
   d) not relevant for estheticians

   a

4. The basic unit of matter is the:
   a) element   c) base
   b) proton   d) atom

   a

5. Electrons:
   a) travel in more than one energy level
   b) have a negative charge
   c) orbit the nucleus of an atom
   d) all of the above are correct

   d

6. All atoms need to:
    a) stay unattached   c) shed excess protons
    b) have a full outer energy level   d) be unstable

    b

7. When negatively and positively charged atoms are attracted to each other, the bond is called:
    a) an ionic bond   c) a biochemical bond
    b) a covalent bond   d) an atomic bond

    a

8. Performance ingredients are sometimes mistakenly called:
    a) active agents   c) active ingredients
    b) active principals   d) key ingredients

    c

9. The FDA requires that cosmetic labels include:
    a) the amount of product in the container
    b) an expiration date
    c) potential allergens or skin irritants
    d) none of the above are correct

    d

10. An emulsion is:
    a) a very refined solution
    b) a heterogeneous diffusion of fat and water
    c) a permanent mixture of two immiscible substances with the aid of an emulsifier
    d) a compound

    c

11. The main ingredient of a water-in-oil emulsion is:
    a) water   c) baking soda
    b) oil   d) lecithin

    b

12. Mineral oil and petrolatum:
    a) come from the earth
    b) protect against dehydration by occlusion
    c) are noncomedogenic
    d) all of the above are correct

    d

13. Plant oils that are less comedogenic are:
    a) coconut oil and sunflower oil
    b) palm oil and jojoba oil
    c) safflower and jojoba oil
    d) coconut oil and palm oil

    c

14. Fatty esters:
    a) are derived from fatty acids and alcohols
    b) almost always end in a-t-e on ingredients labels
    c) a and b are correct
    d) neither a nor b is correct

    C

15. This type of cosmetic ingredient is highly comedogenic:
    a) moisturizers   c) emulsions
    b) emollients   d) plant oils

    b

16. To ensure a product is noncomedogenic:
    a) look for a noncomedogenic claim on the label
    b) ask the salesperson
    c) ask product manufacturers about their testing process
    d) ask your clients how their skin reacts

    C

17. Chemicals that reduce the surface tension between the skin's
    surface and the product are called:
    a) silicones   c) cleansers
    b) emollients   d) surfactants

    d

18. Emulsifiers serve the purpose of:
    a) moisturizing the skin
    b) keeping oils and water blended in a product
    c) keeping oils and water separate in a product
    d) none of the above are correct

    b

19. Cleansing milks can be used by clients with:
    a) sensitive skin   c) dry skin
    b) oilier skin   d) all of the above are correct

    d

20. The acid mantle:
    a) is a protective barrier on the surface of the skin formed by sebum and
       sweat
    b) varies in pH between 4.5 and 6.2
    c) a and b are correct
    d) neither a nor b is corre

    C

21. Fragrances from plant oils:
    a) are especially popular
    b) are called essential oils when they are highly concentrated
    c) never cause allergic reactions
    d) a and b are correct

    d

22. Antioxidants in cosmetics:
    a) are strictly functional ingredients
    b) can help improve the condition of the skin
    c) are not considered preservatives
    d) are strictly performance ingredients

    b

23. The function of a moisturizer is to:
    a) prevent dehydration of the skin
    b) remove traces of makeup and sebum from the skin
    c) help active substances penetrate into the skin
    d) reduce the amount of oil in the skin

    a

24. An ingredient of face masks that has strong absorbent
    properties is:
    a) kaolin   c) calamine
    b) magnesium sulfate   d) rose water

    a

25. The simplest form of chemical is:
    a) an atom   c) a molecule
    b) an element   d) a compound

    b

26. The smallest possible part of an element is:
    a) an atom   c) a compound
    b) a molecule   d) a nucleus

    a

27. Grapeseed extract:
    a) is an antioxidant   c) calms inflammation
    b) is best for sensitive skin   d) all of the above are correct

    d

28. The chemical term for Vitamin C ester is:
    a) ascorbyl palmitate   c) AHAs
    b) ester C   d) Niacin

    a

29. Biochemistry is the study of:
    a) biology and its relation to chemistry
    b) the similarities in biological and chemical reactions
    c) chemical reactions that occur within a living organism
    d) biological reactions that occur within atoms

    c

30. A D&C color is:
    a) inorganic
    b) more intense than other color agents
    c) made from minerals
    d) a and b are correct

    d

31. An example of a compound is:
    a) iron
    c) sodium
    b) water
    d) neon

    b

32. Rust is described as:
    a) an atom
    c) a compound
    b) a molecule
    d) electrons

    c

33. The nucleus of an atom is made up of:
    a) protons and neutrons
    c) neutrons and electrons
    b) protons and electrons
    d) neutrons only

    a

34. The energy level of an atom refers to:
    a) the speed at which the electrons orbit the nucleus
    b) the speed at which the neutrons orbit the nucleus
    c) the orbits in which the electrons travel
    d) the number of electrons in each orbit

    c

35. The valence shell of an atom will be full with:
    a) two electrons
    b) eight electrons
    c) eighteen electrons
    d) an infinite number of electrons

    b

36. Free radicals are related to unstable atoms of:
    a) ozone
    c) oxygen
    b) hydrogen
    d) carbon dioxide

    c

37. Free radicals in the body tend to attack the:
    a) connective tissue in the body
    c) bones
    b) lung cells
    d) lipid cell membrane

    d

38. An example of a functional ingredient is:
    a) beeswax
    c) lipids
    b) glycerin
    d) alpha hydroxy acids

    a

39. Ingredients that cause the skin's surface to change are termed:
    a) functional ingredients
    c) cosmeceuticals
    b) performance ingredients
    d) cosmetics

    b

40. Functional ingredients are also known as:
    a) active ingredients
    b) active principals
    c) cosmeceuticals
    d) product base

     d

41. Ingredients must be listed on the label in order starting with:
    a) an alphabetical descent from A to Z
    b) ingredients with the lowest concentration and ending with the highest
    c) ingredients that are not allergy-tested first, with non-irritating products last
    d) ingredients with the highest concentration, and ending with those with the lowest concentration

    d

42. The most frequently used cosmetic ingredient is:
    a) water
    b) oxygen
    c) lipids
    d) vitamin C

    a

43. A water-in-oil emulsion is:
    a) the most common type of emulsion
    b) of a heavier consistency
    c) anhydrous
    d) suitable for acne skin

    b

44. An anhydrous product:
    a) is designed for very dry skin
    b) does not contain any oil
    c) is a cleanser
    d) is designed for oily and combination skin

    a

Chapter 20

ADVANCED INGREDIENT TECHNOLOGY

1. Which products are the result of new skin care technology?
   - a) serums
   - b) glycoproteins
   - c) polymers
   - d) all of the above are correct   *d*

2. According to the FDA's Cosmetic Act of 1938, cosmetics are NOT intended to:
   - a) alter the appearance
   - b) affect the structures of the body
   - c) promote attractiveness
   - d) cleanse or beautify   *b*

3. Which statement is a cosmetic claim?
   - a) This cream will make your skin younger.
   - b) This cream will make your skin younger-looking.
   - c) a and b are correct
   - d) neither a nor b is correct   *b*

4. A proposed new FDA category is:
   - a) cosmetic
   - b) polymer
   - c) cosmeceutical
   - d) all of the above are correct   *C*

5. Which is a difference between serums and ampoules:
   - a) ampoules are for long-term use
   - b) serums are for long-term use
   - c) ampoules are more user-friendly than serums
   - d) serums are more active than ampoules   *b*

6. Often the most expensive item in a skin care line is:
   a) cleanser
   b) moisturizer
   c) freshener
   d) serum

   d

7. Strategies for selling serums include:
   a) selling them as the most beneficial product
   b) using the serums yourself
   c) including serums in the home care plan
   d) all of the above are correct

   d

8. Which are smaller, thinner liposomes, capable of holding more performance ingredients?
   a) nanosomes
   b) microsponges
   c) polymers
   d) glycoproteins

   a

9. Adjusting your attitude toward selling retail products requires coming to terms with:
   a) selling retail is no different than selling services
   b) recommending and providing quality skin care products is a professional responsibility
   c) a and b are correct
   d) neither a nor b is correct

   C

10. Products that stimulate cell metabolism include:
    a) microsponges
    b) polymers
    c) polyglucans
    d) serums

    C

11. Which antioxidant strengthens capillary networks and increases energy to epidermal cells?
    a) coenzyme Q10
    b) glycoprotein
    c) revitalin-BT
    d) TRF

    a

12. Which helps to strengthen the immune system?
    a) TRF
    b) beta-glucans
    c) glycoproteins
    d) microsponges

    b

13. Which is/are NOT derived from yeast cells?
    a) TRF
    b) poly-glucans
    c) glycoproteins
    d) coenzyme Q10

    d

14. Which enhances cellular metabolism and strengthens skin's natural ability to protect itself from damaging environmental influences?
    a) TRF
    b) polyglucans
    c) glycoproteins
    d) coenzyme Q10

    _C_

15. Which is another term for polymer?
    a) microsponge
    b) glycoprotein
    c) polyglucan
    d) none of the above are correct

    _a_

Chapter *21*

AGING SKIN: MORPHOLOGY AND TREATMENT

1 Intrinsic aging refers to:
   a) sun damage   c) genetic characteristics
   b) lack of proper nutrition   d) multiple wrinkles

C

2. Rhytids is:
   a) the medical term for inflammation of the nose
   b) the medical term for wrinkles
   c) a deficiency of vitamin D
   d) one of the organelles thats produce protein

B

3. Browtosis is:
   a) lack of elasticity in the eyelids
   b) excessive perspiration
   c) a small subdivision of the bronchi
   d) a watery blister

A

4. The histological changes in the skin due to aging occur mainly:
   a) in the epidermis   c) in the muscles
   b) in the subcutaneous layer d) in the dermis

D

5. Dermatoheliosis is:
   a) the technical term for sun-induced aging symptoms
   b) the medical term for inflammation of the skin
   c) a fungal infection of the skin
   d) a generic term for skin diseases

A

6. Ultraviolet B or UVB rays:
   a) are harmless
   b) are longer than UVA rays in the UV spectrum
   c) penetrate into the dermis
   d) are reflected from the lower epidermis

D

7. What is tanning?
   a) a defense mechanism
   b) an aging process
   c) a brown powder obtained from oak galls
   d) a beautiful cosmetic color obtained from the sun

   A

8. Ultraviolet A or UVA rays:
   a) are reflected from the epidermis
   b) are responsible for sunburn
   c) penetrate into the dermis
   d) are shorter than UVB rays

   C

9. What is Polymorphous Light Eruption (PLE)?
   a) sun poisoning
   b) hives associated with sun exposure
   c) freckles and pigmented spots
   d) hypopigmentation

   A

10. What are telangiectasia?
    a) broken capillaries
    b) Greek for hyperpigmentation
    c) dilated blood vessels
    d) none of the above are correct

    C

11. What ingredients should be used by the esthetician to treat telangiectasia?
    a) vitamin K and bioflavonoids   c) hyaluronic acid
    b) chamomile and azulene   d) hydroquinone

    A

12. What is solar elastosis?
    a) elasticity created by the sun
    b) thermonuclear reactions in the sun
    c) sagging of the skin
    d) a lack of elasticity in the soles of the feet

    C

13. How should the esthetician treat seborrheic and actinic keratosis?
    a) refer the client to a dermatologist
    b) remove them with a small razor blade
    c) carefully remove them with lancets
    d) peel with microdermabrasion

    A

14. What are free radicals?
    a) free hydrogen ions in a solution
    b) free hydroxide ions in a solution
    c) unstable molecules or atoms
    d) electron flow

    C
    _____

15. What is crosslinking?
    a) wrinkling in crossed patterns
    b) when free radicals attack the collagen
    c) an inflammation not visually seen
    d) damage of the membrane

    B
    _____

16. What is or are erythema?
    a) red blood cells
    b) female hormones
    c) the end of a long bone
    d) redness in the skin

    D
    _____

17. The Sun Protection Factor (SPF) is:
    a) a number that indicates the shelf life of a product
    b) a number that indicates how long skin can be exposed to the sun
       without burning
    c) the cloudy coverage of the sky
    d) the amount of ozone in the air

    B
    _____

18. One of the best UVA sunscreens is:
    a) octyl methoxycinnimate
    b) zinc oxide
    c) para-aminobenzoic acid (PABA)
    d) salicylic acid

    B
    _____

19. Which SPF is best on a daily basis?
    a) SPF 15
    b) SPF 20
    c) SPF 30
    d) no sun protection is
       needed on a daily basis

    A
    _____

20. Tanning beds and tanning booths:
    a) are safe alternatives to the sun
    b) are beneficial for pre-tanning prior to vacation
    c) use UVB rays only
    d) use UVA rays to tan the skin

    D
    _____

21. The first thing you notice when analyzing sun-damaged skin is:
    a) comedones
    b) coloring and pigmentation
    c) cold sores
    d) oily skin

    B
    _____

22. Without a Wood's lamp the esthetician cannot detect:
    a) hidden hyperpigmentation   c) wrinkles
    b) tactile roughness   d) telangiectasia

    A

23. What are signs of possible skin cancer?
    a) new abnormal-looking growths
    b) a small rough area that bleeds suddenly
    c) lesions that do not heal
    d) all of the above are correct

    D

24. Which is the most serious and deadly form of skin cancer?
    a) melanoma   c) cicatricial carcinoma
    b) basal cell carcinoma   d) squamous cell carcinoma

    A

25. What are the major characteristics used to detect possible melanoma in a lesion?
    a) asymmetry and border   c) diameter
    b) color   d) all of the above are correct

    D

26. Vitamin C and vitamin E are:
    a) vitamins needed to strengthen the nervous system
    b) antioxidants
    c) vitamins needed to strengthen capillary walls
    d) vitamins to protect from virus infections

    B

27. How can we protect the barrier function of the skin?
    a) avoid sun exposure
    b) avoid environmental exposure to cold, heat, wind, and drying soaps
    c) application of emollients and lipids
    d) all of the above are correct

    D

28. How do alpha hydroxy acids (AHAs) help to reverse the signs of sun damage?
    a) by peeling off dead cells
    b) they relayer the epidermis cells
    c) they are good moisturizers
    d) they provide the skin with emollients

    B

29. What are the benefits of paraffin masks for the skin?
    a) they cause nutrients applied under the mask to penetrate deeper
    b) they are warm and cozy
    c) they firm the tissues
    d) they remove wrinkles

    A

30. Which is a contraindication of using thermal masks?
    a) dry skin
    c) mature skin
    b) claustrophobia
    d) sun-damaged skin

    B

31. What is the difference between paraffin masks and thermal masks?
    a) thermal masks are not as hot as paraffin masks
    b) thermal masks make the ingredients penetrate deeper
    c) paraffin masks are applied hot, whereas thermal masks create a heating effect on the skin
    d) paraffin masks can be used on acne skin, whereas thermal masks cannot be used on acne skin

    C

32. What is Pycnogenol?
    a) an antioxidant
    c) a and b are correct
    b) maritime pine bark extract
    d) neither a nor b is correct

    C

33. What is photoaging?
    a) aging with the evidence of photographs
    b) aging symptoms related to sun exposure
    c) aging of photographs
    d) aging of photons

    B

34. What is senile purpura?
    a) easy bruising of the skin
    c) a purple nose with swelling
    b) purple skin with pustules
    d) itching of the skin

    A

35. Expression lines are:
    a) wrinkles due to sun exposure
    b) depressions from muscle movement
    c) lines from pressing on the face
    d) collagen fibers that run in one direction

    B

36. What effect has estrogen on the skin?
    a) responsible for collagen production
    b) increases production of moisture
    c) reduces the activity of sebaceous glands
    d) all of the above are correct

    D

37. What is usually the first sign of premature aging related to sun exposure?
    a) wrinkles
    c) solar urticaria
    b) hyperpigmentation
    d) melanoma

    B

38. What is melasma?
    a) hyperpigmentation
    b) the liquid part of the blood
    c) hypopigmentation
    d) the jellylike liquid between the cells

    A

39. What are nasalabial folds?
    a) folds in the earth eruption found by NASA
    b) little wrinkles in the lips
    c) the folds in the eye lids
    d) expression lines

    D

40. Extrinsic aging refers to:
    a) elastosis due to gravity
    b) premature aging
    c) wrinkles caused by pressures during sleep
    d) genetic characteristics

    B

41. Where do histological changes occur as the skin gets older?
    a) in the dermis
    b) in the epidermis
    c) in the subcutaneous layer
    d) in muscle tissue

    A

42. Where is the moisture held in the epidermis?
    a) in the papillary layer
    b) in the reticulary layer
    c) in the intercellular lipids
    d) in the fatty cells

    C

43. What percentage of collagen does the skin lose per year, beginning in the mid-twenties?
    a) 0%
    b) 1%
    c) 3%
    d) 5%

    B

44. What is actinic damage?
    a) short and severe damage
    b) damage due to clear family history
    c) damage with pustules and papules
    d) damage associated with sun exposure

    D

45. How do you treat sunburned skin in the treatment room?
    a) sunburned skin should not be treated
    b) apply heavy moisturizers
    c) with a basic facial only
    d) apply oil

    A

46. Hives associated with sun exposure are called:
    a) Polymorphous Light Eruption   c) actinic damage
    b) dermatoheliosis   d) solar urticaria

    D

47. What are solar comedones?
    a) comedones on the soles of the feet
    b) comedones caused by sun damage
    c) sun damage that looks like comedones but are not
    d) comedones pertaining to the body

    B

48. What is the best time to go into the sun?
    a) between the hours of 10 am and 3 pm
    b) between the hours of 8 am and 12 pm
    c) early morning or late afternoon
    d) late morning or early afternoon

    C

49. Which of the following statements is correct?
    a) Any tan from sun is an indication of damage to the cells.
    b) You will have to bathe in direct sunlight to receive damaging rays.
    c) Rain clouds filter all of the UV rays.
    d) Dry skin is the main effect of the sun to the skin.

    A

50. Which of the following statements is correct?
    a) UV damage to the eyes can be prevented with a product containing titanium dioxide.
    b) Umbrellas and hats are good substitutes for a broad-spectrum sunscreen.
    c) Apply sunscreen 90 minutes prior to going in direct sunlight.
    d) When in direct sunlight, sunscreen has to be reapplied every 90 minutes.

    D

Chapter 22

SENSITIVE SKIN: MORPHOLOGY AND TREATMENT

1. The skin's natural barrier is made up of:
   a) keratinocytes
   b) lipids
   c) telangiectasias
   d) urticaria

   B

2. The slight redness that shows under a magnifying lamp when examining sensitive skin is:
   a) blood
   b) transepidermal water loss
   c) histamine
   d) pruritis

   A

3. Which is a technique for testing sensitive skin?
   a) dermatographism
   b) enzyme treatment
   c) touch-blanching
   d) microdermabrasion

   C

4. Which is NOT a definitive sign of sensitive skin?
   a) easily sunburned
   b) thinness of skin
   c) history of reactivity
   d) distended capillaries

   D

5. Which of the following best describes dermatographism?
   a) blood vessels are dilated
   b) skin swells easily
   c) skin burns easily
   d) diffuse redness

   B

6. What should you avoid for clients with dermatographic skin?
   a) aloe vera
   b) hydration fluid
   c) microdermabrasion
   d) cryoglobes

   C

7. Individuals with dermatographic skin often have a history of:
   a) asthma
   b) hydroquinone
   c) benzophenone-3
   d) diazolidinyl urea

   A

8. Rashes, redness, and swelling are objective symptoms, which means they are:
   a) environmental factors
   b) visible
   c) itching, burning, or stinging
   d) mechanical irritations

   B

9. Sensitive skin may be more subject to pain than normal skin because:
   a) the skin is erythematic
   b) it is more likely to have allergic reactions
   c) it has barrier guards
   d) nerve endings are closer to the surface

   D

10. As a general rule for sensitive skin, the more products used:
    a) the better to determine an aggravating factor if the client has a problem
    b) the harder to determine an aggravating factor if the client has a problem
    c) the easier to determine whether a product has been tested for irritancy
    d) the more likely a particular product can be identified as 100% nonallergenic

    B

11. An injured or absent barrier function indicates what kind of damage?
    a) exfoliation
    b) edema
    c) erythema
    d) environmental

    D

12. Which of the following statements is true?
    a) An irritant reaction affects only certain individuals.
    b) An allergic reaction affects only certain individuals.
    c) An irritant reaction tends to be more widespread across the skin.
    d) An allergic reaction happens more quickly than an irritant reaction.

    B

13. Redness and flaking caused by overuse of benzoyl peroxide is an example of:
    a) an irritant reaction
    b) an allergic reaction
    c) the immune system rejecting the ingredients
    d) the dermis being exposed

    A

14. In certain people, the immune system will always react when it senses the presence of:
    a) a substance
    b) an irritant
    c) an allergen
    d) barrier function damage

    C

15. The first step in treating skin reactions when you can't determine the offending product is to:
    a) begin enzyme treatments
    b) recommend using fragrance-free products
    c) refer the client to a dermatologist
    d) discontinue all products until the skin clears

    D
    ___

16. What should be used to cool the skin and reduce inflammation caused by irritants?
    a) water compresses   c) antihistamine
    b) topical hydrocortisone   d) stimulating treatments

    A
    ___

17. Which of the following may be used to treat an allergic reaction?
    a) essential oils   c) resorcinol
    b) topical hydrocortisone   d) lanolin

    B
    ___

18. Which of the following statements about allergic reactions is false?
    a) The entire body can be affected.
    b) The reaction can take several days to appear.
    c) The reaction will occur with the first exposure to a particular product or chemical.
    d) The reaction is caused when the immune system rejects a particular substance.

    C
    ___

19. Reactions that result from abrasives such as a scrub or microdermabrasion are:
    a) hereditary   c) mechanical
    b) allergic   d) dermatographic

    C
    ___

20. Which of the following causes an irritant reaction in sensitive skin?
    a) using a particular substance that has been rejected by the person's immune system
    b) using a chemical that burns or overexfoliates the person's skin
    c) removing an ingredient or a product from a client's skin care program
    d) discontinuing all products from a client's skin care program

    B
    ___

21. Of the following frequent cosmetic allergens, which is an emollient?
    a) benzoyl peroxide   c) DMDM hydantoin
    b) lanolin   d) benzophenone-3

    B
    ___

22. Which of the following cosmetic ingredients is NOT a preservative?
    a) paraphenylenediamine
    c) parabens
    b) imidazolidinyl urea
    d) quaternium 15

    A

23. Which of the following statements about rosacea is NOT true?
    a) Rosacea is hereditary.
    b) Rosacea most often affects people with lighter skin.
    c) Rosacea presents as diffuse redness and other skin disorders.
    d) Rosacea is a form of acne.

    D

24. One of the first signs of rosacea is:
    a) a red nose
    b) the skin is sensitive to heat, cold, and possibly touch
    c) blisters and areas of rawness
    d) edema

    A

25. Regarding rosacea, one thing that spicy foods, alcohol, heat, sun, and exercise have in common is that they are:
    a) high pHs
    c) surfactants
    b) vasodilators
    d) vascular irritants

    B

26. If a client with sensitive skin has reservations about treatment, you should first:
    a) suggest products that you think are safe for sensitive skin
    b) start treatment with the fastest-penetrating cleanser
    c) begin aggressive treatment to identify which ingredients seem to work best
    d) discuss the client's experiences and what has and has not worked in the past

    D

27. Which of the following is NOT true of sensitive skin?
    a) The skin is thin and fragile.
    b) The skin has distended capillaries.
    c) Nerve endings and blood vessels are closer to the surface.
    d) Products applied to the skin penetrate quickly.

    B

28. When cleaning sensitive skin, the less foam in the product the better because:
    a) Products with foam are not lab tested.
    b) Foam-free products are made especially for sensitive skin.
    c) The more foam, the more detergent, so more lipids are removed in the process.
    d) Foam products have more oil, which may irritate sensitive skin.

    C

29. The barrier function on sensitive skin can be reinforced with:
    a) heat   c) sunscreen
    b) hot steam   d) lipid ingredients

    D

30. Restoration of the barrier function allows the skin to:
    a) return to a normal, nonirritated state
    b) absorb skin products faster
    c) avoid irritant reactions
    d) have transient sensitivity

    A

31. What do barrier guards, such as petrolatum, do to skin?
    a) help determine the amount of detergent in it
    b) help seal it
    c) increase absorption of possible irritants
    d) further impair the barrier function

    B

32. During salon treatments, what should you use on sensitive skin
    instead of hot steam?
    a) cool steam   c) hot water
    b) no steam   d) heat

    A

33. Sensitive skin is more tolerant of which two sunscreen agents:
    a) benzophenone-3 and paraminobenzoic acid
    b) borage and evening primrose
    c) phospholipids and linoleic acid
    d) zinc oxide and titanium dioxide

    D

34. Why are sunscreens with zinc oxide and titanium dioxide better
    for sensitive skin?
    a) They absorb sunlight, decreasing the amount of heat reflected on the
       skin.
    b) They reflect sunlight, decreasing the amount of heat absorbed by the
       skin.
    c) They lower transepidermal water loss.
    d) They keep harmful bacteria out of sunscreen products.

    B

35. Why are high SPF sunscreens more likely to irritate sensitive
    skin?
    a) they stimulate nerve endings in the dermis
    b) they decrease the skin's hydration level
    c) they contain more absorbing chemicals
    d) they thin an already poor barrier

    C

36. Which of the following statements is FALSE?
    a) On sensitive skin, alpha hydroxy acids may thin an already poor barrier.
    b) If the barrier function is impaired, low-pH acids can cause irritation.
    c) Some sunscreens can be both reflective and absorbing.
    d) Exfoliating agents can be used safely on any skin type.

    D

37. Why should products for sensitive skin be fragrance-free?
    a) Fragrance is a major cause of cosmetic allergy.
    b) Fragrance is a major cosmetic irritant.
    c) Fragrances dehydrate the skin.
    d) Fragrances absorb heat and sunlight.

    A

38. Which one of the following is important to the efficacy of a skin care product?
    a) essential oils
    b) preservatives
    c) color agents
    d) fragrance

    B

39. Which preservative works by releasing small amounts of formaldehyde?
    a) resorcinal
    b) benzoyl peroxide
    c) formalin-releasers
    d) hydroquinone

    C

40. Which of the following is NOT recommended when treating sensitive skin?
    a) using a nonfragranced, nonfoaming cleansing milk with a soothing agent
    b) using a soft sponge, applying the cleanser directly to the face
    c) using your fingertips to massage the cleansing lotion across the skin
    d) removing the cleanser using cool, wet cotton pads or cloths

    B

41. A facial massage on sensitive skin should be limited to how many minutes:
    a) 3 to 5 minutes
    b) 5 to 10 minutes
    c) 8 to 10 minutes
    d) 20 to 30 minutes

    B

42. Which is a term for a small plastic or glass container that holds refrigerant fluid?
    a) a Lucas device
    b) effleurage
    c) cryoglobe
    d) formalin-releaser

    C

43. For home care, gel masks are recommended for sensitive skin
    because they:
    a) are alcohol free
    b) are fragrance free
    c) contain humectants
    d) do not dry or tighten the skin _____ D

44. Salon treatments for sensitive skin should be:
    a) ice cold
    b) room temperature
    c) warm
    d) hot _____ B

45. Which statement is NOT true for people with sensitive skin?
    a) They often have impaired barrier function.
    b) They often have reduced lipid production.
    c) They are more susceptible to allergens and irritants.
    d) They require a complex treatment regimen initially to identify
       sensitivities. _____ D

Chapter 23

HYPERPIGMENTATION: MORPHOLOGY AND TREATMENT

1. Which of the following forms of hyperpigmentation is the very first sign of sun-induced skin damage?
   a) melasma
   b) chloasma
   c) mottling
   d) inflammation

   C

2. Which of the following forms of hyperpigmentation typically appears as a "pregnancy mask"?
   a) mottling
   b) acne excorieé
   c) chloasma
   d) melasma

   D

3. The major cause of hyperpigmentation is:
   a) elastosis
   b) sun exposure
   c) actinic keratoses
   d) hormone fluctuations

   B

4. Hyperpigmentation occurs because of an overproduction of:
   a) melanocytes
   b) hormones
   c) hydroxy acids
   d) melanin

   D

5. Hyperpigmented clients should avoid exposure to sunlight and:
   a) hydroquinone
   b) heat
   c) zinc oxide
   d) alpha hydroxy acid

   B

6. The problem of hyperpigmentation is LEAST prominent among the following groups:
   a) Hispanics
   b) Asians
   c) Caucasians
   d) individuals of African descent

   C

7. Postinflammatory hyperpigmentation (PIH) can be caused by:
   a) alpha hydroxy acids
   b) mottling
   c) zinc oxide
   d) sunscreens

   A

8. How often should hyperpigmentation clients use AHAs and other exfoliating agents on their problem areas?
   a) weekly
   b) twice weekly
   c) daily
   d) monthly

   C

9. Hyperpigmentation should be treated with AHA in a concentration of:
   a) 0.5% - 1.5%
   b) 3% - 5%
   c) 15% - 20%
   d) 8% - 10%

   D

10. AHAs work to treat hyperpigmentation by:
    a) blocking the sun's UV rays
    b) removing keratinocytes that contain melanin
    c) suppressing melanocyte activity
    d) regulating hormone levels in the skin

    B

11. Which of the following is the only agent approved by the FDA for bleaching or fading melanin?
    a) alpha hydroxy acid
    b) beta hydroxy acid
    c) hydroquinone
    d) titanium dioxide

    C

12. What is the maximum concentration of hydroquinone in over-the-counter formulations?
    a) 2%
    b) 7%
    c) 4%
    d) 0.05%

    A

13. To accelerate the lightening process, physicians often use hydroquinone in combination with:
    a) azelaic acid
    b) magnesium ascorbyl phosphate
    c) tretinoin
    d) ascorbyl glucosamine

    C

14. Salon treatments for hyperpigmentation usually begin with:
    a) a series of phototherapy sessions
    b) application of hydrators and skin toners
    c) microdermabrasion
    d) an AHA series

    D

15. What is the maximum suggested AHA concentration for a salon-administered AHA series?

    a) 30%   c) 25%
    b) 15%   d) 50%

16. Which of the following procedures should be reserved for non-responsive cases of hyperpigmentation?

    a) AHA series   c) resorcinol exfoliations
    b) salicylic acid treatments d) mechanical abrasions

    C

Chapter 24

ACNE: MORPHOLOGY AND TREATMENT

1. Which of the following is NOT a cause of acne?
   a) hormones
   b) heredity
   c) retention hyperkeratosis
   d) dirt

   D

2. The waxy substance that coats follicular cell buildup and leads to additional cell buildup is known as:
   a) pus
   b) sebum
   c) oil
   d) *p. acnes*

   B

3. A plug of oil and sebum inside the follicle is known as a:
   a) pustule
   b) pock
   c) comedo
   d) lipid

   C

4. Open comedones are also known as:
   a) blackheads
   b) whiteheads
   c) pustules
   d) cysts

   A

5. What causes the darkening of the sebaceous material in blackheads?
   a) infection
   b) inflammation
   c) oxidation
   d) dirt

   C

6. Closed comedones are also known as:
   a) blackheads
   b) whiteheads
   c) pustules
   d) cysts

   B

7. The acne bacteria *p. acnes* are anaerobic, which means:
   a) they reside deep within the skin
   b) they are highly active and replicate quickly
   c) they cannot survive when exposed to oxygen
   d) they are extremely small and mobile

   c

8. Open and closed comedones are known as noninflammatory acne lesions, which means they are NOT:
   a) infectious   c) contagious
   b) oily   d) red or inflamed

   D

9. *Propionibacterium acnes* bacteria grow within the follicle because they feed off:
   a) leukocytes   c) oil
   b) pus   d) sebum

   B

10. Which of the following is NOT part of the debris that spills out of a ruptured follicle?
    a) dead cells   c) bacteria
    b) leukocytes   d) sebum

    B

11. An inflammatory acne lesion is also known as:
    a) an acne cyst   c) a pustule
    b) an acne papule   d) an open comedone

    B

12. An elevated red lesion with a white center is a:
    a) pustule   c) pock
    b) papule   d) cyst

    A

13. The noninflammatory lesion that most often leads to papule or pustule formation is the:
    a) open comedo   c) closed comedo
    b) blackhead   d) nodule

    C

14. Nodules are palpable, which means they:
    a) contain pus and bacteria
    b) are filled with sebaceous material
    c) are surrounded by leukocytes
    d) can be felt or palpated easily under the skin

    D

Brandon R

I LOVE YOU

15. Cysts are formed when:
    a) sebum and oil coat the follicle
    b) open comedones burst
    c) the skin forms hardened tissue to halt the spread of bacterial infection
    d) oxidation occurs in the follicle   *C*

16. Cystic acne does NOT respond to surface esthetic treatment because:
    a) the *p. acnes* bacteria are too numerous
    b) leukocytes have blocked too many follicles
    c) sebum plugs have become over-impacted
    d) the cysts and nodules are too deep to be reached by
       surface treatment   *D*

17. Clients with cystic acne should be:
    a) given multiple surface treatments
    b) treated with astringent and toner
    c) referred to a dermatologist
    d) instructed to change their dietary habits   *C*

18. Sebaceous filaments are also called:
    a) microcomedones   c) open comedones
    b) clogged pores   d) follicles   *B*

19. What is the main difference between sebaceous filaments and open comedones?
    a) Sebaceous filaments contain pus, open comedones do not.
    b) Sebaceous filaments appear in the T-zone of oily skin, open comedones do not.
    c) Sebaceous filaments are likely to become pustules, open comedones are not.
    d) Sebaceous filaments contain primarily just sebaceous secretions, while open comedones have a build up of dead cells mixed with the sebum.   *D*

20. Sebaceous filaments are difficult to control but can be treated with:
    a) soap and water   c) hydroquinone
    b) alpha hydroxy acid   d) azelaic acid   *B*

21. Which of the following stimulates the sebaceous gland to produce sebum?
    a) hydroquinone   c) alpha hydroxy acid
    b) dihydrotestosterone   d) *propionibacterium acnes*   *B*

22. As sebum begins flowing through the follicle, the follicle walls
    tend to:
    a) become brittle   c) dissolve
    b) contract   d) stretch   D

23. Small comedones may appear on facial skin as early as age:
    a) 3   c) 10
    b) 5   d) 12   C

24. Treating acne in very young clients is often difficult because very
    young clients:
    a) have smaller, tougher comedones
    b) lack the discipline necessary to follow treatment instructions
    c) have higher *p. acnes* counts
    d) have heavier sebum flow   B

25. Which of the following is NOT recommended for teenagers try-
    ing to control pimples?
    a) dihydrotestoterone   c) sunscreen formulated for oily skin
    b) alpha hydroxy acid gel d) foaming cleanser   A

26. Women who never had acne as teenagers may experience
    chronic breakout problems later in life in a condition known as:
    a) cystic acne   c) premenstrual acne
    b) retention hyperkeratosis d) aerobic acne   C

27. Premenstrual acne, a hormonal acne, most often affects this
    portion of the face:
    a) forehead   c) cheeks
    b) nose   d) chin   D

28. The most common form of acne is known as:
    a) cystic acne   c) premenstrual acne
    b) aerobic acne   d) comedonal acne   B D

29. Inflammatory acne is caused by:
    a) a sudden decrease in sebum production
    b) follicular comedones
    c) a surge in sebum production
    d) multiple papules   B C

30. Cosmetics and skin care products that can inflame the follicle are referred to as:
    a) caustic
    b) acnegenic
    c) anaerobic
    d) hyperkeratotic

    _B_

31. To control acne-causing hormonal fluctuations in women, a physician might prescribe:
    a) an antibiotic
    b) alpha hydroxy acid
    c) an anti-inflammatory
    d) certain birth control pills

    _D_

32. Which of the following foods is most likely to aggravate acne?
    a) pizza
    b) hamburgers
    c) chocolate
    d) none of the above are correct

    _D_

33. Many cosmetics and skin care products can aggravate acne because they often:
    a) contain high concentrations of *p. acnes* bacteria
    b) contain fatty ingredients that are comedogenic
    c) contain minimal amounts of alpha hydroxy acid
    d) are applied improperly

    _B_

34. A method of categorizing or describing the severity of acne is called:
    a) scaling
    b) measuring
    c) grading
    d) weighting

    _C_

35. Which of the following is NOT true about Grade 1 acne?
    a) it is the most severe grade of acne
    b) it has some closed comedones
    c) it has few papules
    d) it consists mostly of open comedones

    _A_

36. Deep nodules and cysts are characteristic of:
    a) Grade 2 acne
    b) Grade 1 acne
    c) Grade 4 acne
    d) Grade 3 acne

    _C_

37. Clients with Grade 4 acne must be treated:
    a) with foaming cleanser
    b) by an esthetician
    c) with concentrated exfoliants
    d) by a dermatologist

    _D_

38. An esthetician's first step in helping a client manage acne is to:
    a) instruct on changes in dietary habits
    b) perform a deep-pore cleanse
    c) inventory a client's skin products and eliminate comedogenic items
    d) perform an AHA series of exfoliations

    _C_

39. The presence of many closed comedones can be a sign of acne cosmetica, which is:
    a) caused by too much sun exposure
    b) another name for inflammatory acne
    c) one of the most difficult forms of acne to treat
    d) caused or worsened by multiple types of skin and skin-care products

    _D_

40. Oil-free cosmetics are:
    a) always appropriate for acne-prone clients
    b) non-comedogenic
    c) properly tested for comedogenicity
    d) not necessarily non-comedogenic

    _D_

41. Hydrators intended for acne-prone skin should contain:
    a) alpha hydroxy acid   c) lipids
    b) water-binding humectants   d) hydroquinone

    _B_

42. For controlling oily skin, the more aggressive cleansers are usually those that:
    a) contain lipids   c) foam
    b) are used twice a day   d) are clear or white in color

    _C_

43. Which of the following is NOT true about cleansers containing AHAs?
    a) they may also contain benzoyl peroxide
    b) they eliminate the need for AHA treatment after cleansing
    c) they are available in foaming formulations
    d) they may contain salicylic acid

    _B_

44. Which of the following ingredients may be present in toners as an antibacterial agent?
    a) witch hazel   c) sulfur
    b) SD alcohol   d) glycolic acid

    _C_

45. Exfoliating agents are also known as keratolytics, which means they:
    a) dissolve *p. acnes* bacteria
    b) increase the moisture content in keratinocytes
    c) help keratinocytes replicate
    d) dissolve keratin

    D

46. Which of the following is NOT true of AHAs?
    a) the FDA considers them as drugs
    b) they are not antibacterial
    c) they help remove follicular debris
    d) they can be found in foaming cleansers

    A

47. Cleansing of the skin more than three times a day can:
    a) reduce the number of cysts
    b) eliminate the need for AHA gels
    c) cause hormonal fluctuations
    d) trigger acne detergicans

    D

48. Acne can worsen in high humidity because:
    a) perspiration increases in humid conditions
    b) follicles expand in diameter in high humidity
    c) oils evaporate less easily and sebum is more likely to stay on the skin
    d) *p. acnes* bacteria multiply more quickly in moist conditions

    C

49. Stress is a contributing factor to acne because:
    a) diets tend to become unhealthful during times of stress
    b) stress causes hormonal fluctuations
    c) hygiene tends to worsen in stressful times
    d) increases in perspiration occur during times of stress

    B

50. Flat, scraped lesions on a client's skin are a sign of:
    a) hyper-exfoliation   c) acne excorieé
    b) acne cosmetica   d) acne detergicans

    C

51. Redness or tightness of the skin after use of a cleansing agent is a sign that:
    a) the cleanser is working properly
    b) sebum production is under control
    c) the cleanser is not of sufficient strength
    d) the cleanser may be too strong or too harsh

    D

52. During morning home care for acne, AHA exfoliating gel should be applied:
    a) before cleansing
    b) immediately after toning
    c) immediately before toning
    d) after applying sunscreen

    B

53. Exfoliating gels are NOT appropriate for:
    a) teenagers
    b) male clients
    c) clients using prescription keratolytics
    d) clients with premenstrual acne

    C

54. When treating acne excorieé, the esthetician should focus on:
    a) getting the client to stop picking at acne lesions
    b) reducing the hyperpigmentation
    c) administering aggressive exfoliation
    d) instructing dietary changes

    A

55. The only drug routinely effective against acne cysts is:
    a) Retin-A
    b) Differin
    c) Accutane
    d) Benzamycin

    C

56. Which of the following is NOT true about clients who are taking Accutane:
    a) they must have their blood monitored routinely
    b) they should use exfoliating agents regularly
    c) they cannot be waxed anywhere on their bodies
    d) they may experience changes in their blood lipid levels

    B

57. Disincrustation is a process that:
    a) removes dead skin
    b) kills *p. acnes* bacteria
    c) dissolves papules
    d) softens sebum deposits

    D

58. Which of following should NOT be used before or during extraction?
    a) disincrustation product
    b) steam
    c) toner
    d) galvanic current

    C

59. A lancet is used to:
    a) dilate follicles
    b) apply galvanic current
    c) apply pressure to the outside edges of a clogged follicle
    d) puncture and drain pustules

    A

60. Which of the following statements about lancets is NOT true?
    a) they must always be sterile and disposable
    b) they should never puncture the skin
    c) they should be held at a 90-degree angle to the skin
    d) they should be held parallel to the skin

    C

61. After extraction, an esthetician must apply:
    a) an AHA wash   c) hydroquinone
    b) an antiseptic   d) emollients

    B

62. Which of the following is NOT true about high frequency current?
    a) it stimulates blood and lymph flow
    b) it kills bacteria on the skin's surface
    c) it can reduce swelling of pustules and papules
    d) it can shrink deep cysts

    D

63. High frequency zapping or sparking of acne lesions is known as:
    a) galvanization   c) electroextraction
    b) fulguration   d) hyperexfoliation

    B

64. Masks applied to the skin after high frequency treatment should be allowed to dry for:
    a) 3 - 5 minutes   c) 10 - 15 minutes
    b) 5 - 10 minutes   d) 15 - 20 minutes

    C

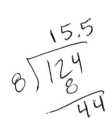

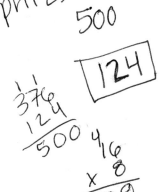

Chapter **25**

ETHNIC SKIN: MORPHOLOGY AND TREATMENT

1. Individuals with fair skin are at higher risk for solar damage and premature aging due to:
   a) ultraviolet radiation
   b) decreased melanin levels
   c) sebaceous glands
   d) hyperkeratosis

   B

2. The purpose of melanin in our skin is to:
   a) prevent the skin from being oily
   b) shed dead skin cells
   c) filter ultraviolet radiation
   d) contribute to the natural shine of the skin

   C

3. Which of the following statements is NOT true?
   a) Ethnic skin has more melanin.
   b) All skin is susceptible to solar damage resulting in premature aging.
   c) The more melanin the skin has, the more damage it can sustain.
   d) Ethnic skin appears resilient but it may require gentle treatments.

   C

4. Which of these is a fallacy about black skin?
   a) Black skin is susceptible to skin damage.
   b) Black skin is oilier than other skin types.
   c) Oil-based creams contribute to the natural shine of black skin.
   d) Black skin has more and larger sebaceous glands.

   B

5. A common problem for black skin is:
   a) hyperkeratosis
   b) reduced melanin
   c) too much hydration
   d) there are only two categories of black skin

   A

6. When skin desquamates, it:
   a) becomes oily
   b) shines
   c) sheds
   d) sweats

   C

7. What accounts for an ashy cast to black skin?
   a) the accumulation of dead skin cells
   b) the exfoliation of dead skin cells
   c) the penetration of ultraviolet radiation
   d) erythema

   A

8. Which statement does NOT explain why black skin is not as prone to skin cancer?
   a) The melanosome produces a higher amount of melanin in black skin.
   b) Black skin has more sudoriferous glands.
   c) Black skin is much thicker than Caucasian skin.
   d) Black skin is better protected from ultraviolet radiation.

   B

9. Which one of the following is black skin NOT prone to having?
   a) leukoderma
   b) vitiligo
   c) melasma
   d) rosacea

   D

10. Which of the following terms does NOT refer to pigmentation?
    a) keloid
    b) melasma
    c) chloasma
    d) leukoderma

    A

11. Which of the following does NOT contribute to hyperpigmentation?
    a) oral contraceptives
    b) aging
    c) hormone replacement therapies
    d) pregnancy

    B

12. Black skin with mild to moderate melasma can be treated with:
    a) exfoliation
    b) azelaic acid and hydroquinone
    c) oil-based creams
    d) slow-releasing enzymes

    B

13. Why must you be extra careful when performing extractions on black skin?
    a) The extracted area can hyperpigment, leaving a darkened mark.
    b) The extracted area can hypopigment, leaving a lightened mark.
    c) The extracted area can become dehydrated.
    d) The extracted area can desquamate.

    A

14. Black skin is highly subject to:
    a) skin cancer
    b) thinning of the epidermis
    c) keloid formation
    d) oiliness

    C

15. How does black skin display erythema in a dermatitis reaction?
    a) The skin loses pigmentation in that area.
    b) The skin turns bluish or purplish.
    c) The skin has an ashy cast.
    d) The skin can be pigmented in a blotchy manner.

    B

16. Scars are formed by:
    a) fibroblastic cells
    b) erythema
    c) melasma
    d) postinflammatory hyperpigmentation

    A

17. Why might aggressive dermabrasion be dangerous on postacne scars on black skin?
    a) It could cause premature aging.
    b) Keloids might form as a result.
    c) It is not a dangerous treatment for postacne scars.
    d) The skin could elasticize.

    B

18. Keloidal tissue may form when fibroblasts continue to deposit what at the wound site?
    a) collagen
    b) melanin
    c) azelaic acid
    d) beta hydroxy acids

    A

19. Black skin can form keloids in response to which of the following?
    a) sun damage
    b) hormonal imbalance
    c) body piercing
    d) ultraviolet radiation

    C

20. How are the protrusions resulting from thickened keloidal tissue treated?
    a) with low concentrations of hydroquinone
    b) by excision
    c) by applying lemon balm extracts
    d) by performing gommage rub-off mechanical exfoliation

    B

21. Instead of harsh dermabrasion, what should you use on post-acne scars on black skin?
    a) a lancet
    b) a comedone extractor
    c) caution
    d) exfoliation

    C

22. Healthy black skin doesn't show the effects of aging as early as Caucasian skin due to:
    a) hyperkeratinized cells
    b) natural pigmentary ultraviolet protection
    c) sebum plugs
    d) photosensitization

    B

23. Which of the following is NOT a melanin-blocking ingredient?
    a) kojic acid   c) alpha hydroxy acid
    b) azeleic acid   d) hydroquinone

    C

24. When using hyperpigmentation products, clients with black skin must avoid:
    a) sun exposure
    b) antiaging and firming treatments
    c) sunscreen and sunblocks
    d) kojic acid

    A

25. Which skin is probably the most sensitive to topical treatments?
    a) Native American   c) black
    b) Caucasian   d) Asian

    D

26. What does Asian skin tend to do when traumatized by aggressive substances?
    a) hyperpigment   c) become splotchy
    b) hypopigment   d) shed

    A

27. Which of the following is NOT recommended for exfoliating Asian skin?
    a) gommage rub-off mechanical exfoliation
    b) low-level AHAs or BHAs
    c) high-level AHAs or BHAs
    d) slow-releasing enzymes

    C

28. What is the most important product an Asian client can use?
    a) melanin blockers   c) BHAs
    b) AHAs   d) sunscreen or sunblock

    D

29. Which of the following is NOT recommended for Asian skin?
    a) lemon balm
    b) magnesium ascorbyl phosphate
    c) bearberry
    d) Retin-A

    D

30. It is recommended that Asians use sunscreens that contain what ingredient?
    a) titanium dioxide
    b) collagen
    c) melanosome
    d) AHAs

    A

31. Which of the following statements about Hispanic and Native American skin is false?
    a) It does not normally sunburn.
    b) It may hyperpigment and develop uneven pigment and splotchiness.
    c) Aggressive AHA or BHA treatments may cause temporary hyperpigmentation.
    d) Hyperpigmentation takes longer to subside than in Asian or black skin.

    D

32. Signs of aging are delayed in Asian skin because of its:
    a) melanin
    b) elastic resiliency
    c) hydration levels
    d) resistance to allergic or irritant reactions

    B

33. Which kind of ethnic skin has the strongest hair growth and root system?
    a) Caucasian
    b) Native American
    c) Hispanic
    d) black

    C

34. Waxing and extractions are often difficult on Hispanic and Native American skin for all of the following reasons EXCEPT:
    a) the skin may be prone to bruising
    b) the skin is prone to dehydration
    c) the skin has a predisposition to pigment around a lesion
    d) the skin is often thicker and has more sebaceous secretions

    B

35. Which is the common denominator in all ethnic skin?
    a) prone to hyperpigmentation
    b) easily bruised
    c) low skin cancer rates
    d) tendency to form keloids

    A

36. In general, what treatment best enhances exfoliation and cleanses impacted follicles in ethnic skin?
    a) applying oil-based creams
    b) dermabrasion
    c) extraction
    d) superficial peels

    D

Chapter 26

EXFOLIATION

1. To desquamate is to:
   a) lighten the skin
   b) remove dead skin cells
   c) remove hair from the skin
   d) remove oily buildup from skin _____ **B**

2. Which of the following is LEAST likely to interfere with skin's natural exfoliation cycle?
   a) hormonal fluctuations
   b) pollution
   c) diet
   d) excessive oil _____ **C**

3. Although it slows with age, skin's average natural cycle of renewal is approximately:
   a) 5 - 7 days
   b) 10 days
   c) 21 days
   d) 28 - 30 days _____ **D**

4. Which of the following is NOT a form of mechanical exfoliation?
   a) gommages
   b) galvanic current
   c) granular scrubs
   d) microdermabrasion _____ **B**

5. Mechanical exfoliation via home scrubs is often recommended:
   a) daily
   b) once a week
   c) once a month
   d) 2 - 3 times per week _____ **D**

6. Alpha hydroxy and beta hydroxy acids (AHAs and BHAs) are examples of:
   a) antibiotics
   b) chemoexfoliants
   c) antioxidants
   d) drying agents _____ **B**

7. Granular scrubs exfoliate via:
   a) disinfection
   b) friction
   c) extraction
   d) chemical reaction _____ **B**

8. In salon exfoliation treatments, granular scrubs are often used with:
   a) galvanic current
   b) high frequency electrodes
   c) the brush machine
   d) hydroquinone

   C

9. Gommage is a French word that means:
   a) erase
   b) exfoliate
   c) desquamate
   d) cleanse

   A

10. Gommages should never be used on clients who have:
    a) acne
    b) rosacea
    c) open comedones
    d) retention hyperkeratosis

    B

11. Steam should NOT be used with a gommage because:
    a) it causes follicles to contract
    b) the additional moisture breeds bacteria
    c) the skin can become overheated
    d) it makes the gommage gummy and difficult to remove

    D

12. Microdermabrasion is similar to:
    a) steam cleaning
    b) pressure washing
    c) sandblasting
    d) paint stripping

    C

13. Any procedure that removes cells beyond the stratum corneum is considered:
    a) an aggressive exfoliation
    b) a medical peeling
    c) microdermabrasion
    d) chemoexfoliation

    B

14. The chemical most often used for medium depth peels is:
    a) resorcinol
    b) azelaic acid
    c) trichloroacetic acid
    d) sulfur

    C

15. Deep peels are performed with phenol, which is:
    a) highly acidic
    b) highly basic
    c) a powerful alkaline
    d) a controlled substance

    A

16. Laser resurfacing surgery is an ablative procedure, which means it:
    a) sanitizes parts of the skin
    b) relaxes the layers of the skin
    c) adds depth to the layers of the skin
    d) removes parts of the skin

    D

17. Which of the following is NOT likely to improve through AHA exfoliations?
    a) clogged pores
    b) hyperpigmentation
    c) cystic acne
    d) rough skin

    C

18. Alpha hydroxy acids work by:
    a) dissolving sebum
    b) loosening chemical bonds between keratinocytes
    c) strengthening lipids in the skin surface
    d) gently burning the stratum corneum

    B

19. The most commonly used AHA in salon treatments is:
    a) salicylic acid
    b) malic acid
    c) glycolic acid
    d) citric acid

    C

20. Which of the following is NOT true about routine AHA use?
    a) it can minimize the appearance of large pores
    b) it can help control oiliness
    c) it can help control formation of microcomedones
    d) it can cure retention hyperkeratosis

    D

21. AHAs can improve hyperpigmentation by removing keratinocytes containing:
    a) sebaceous filaments
    b) melanosomes
    c) desmosomes
    d) melanocytes

    B

22. AHAs can help reduce dehydration by:
    a) removing intercellular lipids
    b) releasing fluids held in keratinocytes
    c) slowing cell renewal rates
    d) stimulating production of intercellular lipids

    D

23. Clients desiring salon AHA treatments should treat themselves at home with AHAs for at least:
    a) 72 hours
    b) one week
    c) two weeks
    d) one month

    C

24. AHA products used for salon treatments should have a pH of not less than:
    a) 2.0
    b) 3.0
    c) 8.0
    d) 10.0

    B

25. Clients using AHAs must also use a sunscreen with an SPF of not less than:
    a) 2
    b) 8
    c) 12
    d) 15

    D

26. Which of following is NOT a drying agent that can be used as a spot treatment on raised pimples?
    a) sulfur-resorcinol
    b) green-tea extract
    c) salicylic acid
    d) benzoyl peroxide

    B

27. When administering salon AHA treatment, the client's head should be slightly elevated to:
    a) make the client more comfortable
    b) prevent the client from getting dizzy
    c) allow the client a better view of the procedure
    d) prevent gel from rolling back into the eye

    D

28. Which portion of the face should the esthetician start with when applying AHA gel?
    a) the cheeks
    b) the chin
    c) the forehead
    d) the nose

    C

29. In applying AHA gel, the esthetician should use:
    a) cotton swabs
    b) cotton pads
    c) hand towels
    d) rubber gloves

    A

30. If the client tells you to remove the AHA product, you should:
    a) ignore the request
    b) reassure the client that any discomfort will pass quickly
    c) remove the product immediately
    d) discuss the client's concerns further

    C

31. Typically, AHA gel should be left on the skin for:
    a) 45 minutes
    b) one hour
    c) 5 minutes
    d) 10 minutes

    D

32. In the first removal step, an esthetician should remove the AHA gel using:
    a) hand towels
    b) a steady stream of water
    c) wet gauze pads
    d) cotton balls soaked in toner

    C

33. Which of the following statements about Jessner's exfoliation is NOT true:
    a) It is much more aggressive than alpha hydroxy acid exfoliation.
    b) It is an excellent first-choice for routine skin conditions.
    c) It can cause skin to flake.
    d) It can cause temporary hyperpigmentation.

    B

34. Jessner's solution is a liquid solution of lactic acid, salicylic acid, and resorcinol in a solvent of:
    a) SD alcohol
    b) isopropyl alcohol
    c) ethanol
    d) water

    C

35. Treatment with Jessner's involves application of a prepping solution, usually:
    a) rubbing alcohol
    b) toner
    c) lactic acid
    d) acetone

    D

36. The appearance of white patches on Jessner's-treated skin is known as:
    a) scaling
    b) flaking
    c) frosting
    d) caking

    C

37. How long does it take for darkened, Jessner's-treated skin to begin peeling?
    a) three to four hours
    b) 24 to 36 hours
    c) two days
    d) three to four days

    D

38. How long must Jessner's-treated clients avoid exposure to the sun?
    a) two weeks
    b) six weeks
    c) one month
    d) six months

    B

39. Which of the following is particularly useful for treating resistant hyperpigmentation?
    a) lactic acid
    b) azelaic acid
    c) resorcinol paste
    d) acetone

    C

40. The most commonly used beta hydroxy acid (BHa) is:
    a) glycolic acid
    b) salicylic acid
    c) trichloroacetic acid
    d) lactic acid

    B

41. BHAs are described as lipophilic, meaning they have the ability to:
    a) increase the lipid content of the epidermis
    b) distribute liposomes throughout skin tissue
    c) restore keratinocytes
    d) dissolve oil

    D

42. In addition to being lipophilic, BHAs can also be:
    a) epidermolytic
    b) analgesic
    c) comedogenic
    d) acnegenic

    B

43. Which of the following is NOT a true statement about salicylic acid?
    a) it can suppress the number of *p. acnes* bacteria
    b) it can damage live cells in large numbers
    c) it can stimulate cell turnover cycles
    d) it can reduce the number of microcomedones

    B

44. Salicylic acid exfoliations should be conducted no more than every:
    a) six to eight weeks
    b) other week
    c) two to four weeks
    d) three weeks

    A

45. Hyperpigmentation after BHA exfoliation is:
    a) a sign of underlying skin damage
    b) an indication that the procedure was performed incorrectly
    c) normal, and is considered a positive development
    d) likely to be permanent

    C

46. When performing a BHA treatment, an esthetician should:
    a) also perform microcomedone extractions
    b) not administer any other treatments
    c) perform soothing, cool steam therapy
    d) apply depilatory as well

    B

47. Before applying the BHA, an esthetician should apply:
    a) a sunscreen with an SPF of 15 or higher
    b) hydrating gel
    c) resorcinol
    d) a complete degreaser

    D

48. During application of the BHA, a client may experience:
   a) chills and numbness   c) intense itching
   b) a warm, prickly sensation   d) temporary shortness of breath   *B*

49. During the BHA treatment, it is recommended that the esthetician:
   a) work quickly and quietly
   b) leave the client alone for several minutes while the product works
   c) tend to other clients receiving similar treatments
   d) speak with the client to keep him or her comfortable   *D*

50. After BHA treatment, application of sunscreen containing titanium dioxide or zinc oxide is recommended because these agents are:
   a) non-comedogenic   c) antibacterial
   b) anti-inflammatory   d) keratolytic   *B*

51. The most common enzymes used in cosmetics are derived from:
   a) fungi   c) fruits or vegetables
   b) bacteria   d) tree bark   *C*

52. Enzymes have a catalytic effect, which means they:
   a) kill harmful bacteria
   b) help clear plugged follicles
   c) slow sebum production
   d) speed up or trigger chemical reactions   *D*

53. The enzyme bromelain comes from:
   a) papaya   c) pineapple
   b) kiwi   d) apricot   *C*

54. Enzyme exfoliating agents are usually packaged in this form:
   a) powder   c) ointment
   b) gel   d) paste   *A*

55. Before using enzyme exfoliants, clients and estheticians should:
   a) discontinue use of sunscreen several days prior to enzyme application
   b) discontinue use of moisturizers several days prior to enzyme treatment
   c) discontinue use of AHAs and BHAs within a few days of enzyme treatments
   d) begin using AHAs up to the time the enzyme exfoliant is applied   *C*

56. When choosing a form of chemical exfoliation, the esthetician should:

    a) always select enzymes because they are naturally derived
    b) use what the client prefers
    c) select the product he or she is most familiar with
    d) try to match the client's skin condition with the procedure most likely to help

    D

Chapter 27

HOLISTIC/ALTERNATIVE SKIN CARE

1. Which best describes the term "holistic" as a treatment method?
   a) the analysis of a system   c) from the inside out
   b) the sum of the individual parts   d) interacting wholes

   D

2. It is thought that holism may have risen over the past few decades due to:
   a) declining respect for Western medicine
   b) increasing medical specialization
   c) the overall desire to focus more on symptoms
   d) the demand for isolating treatments for mind and body

   A

3. Another term for Western medicine is:
   a) homeopathic   c) alternative
   b) allopathic   d) natural

   B

4. Our definition of the word holistic should go beyond skin care to include:
   a) Ayurvedic practices
   b) health care and life in general
   c) allopathic medicine
   d) natural therapies

   B

5. Which course of treatment would be considered truly holistic?
   a) using only natural ingredients
   b) treatments based only on Ayurvedic practices
   c) focusing on the mind, body, and soul combined
   d) a mixture of Western and natural therapies

   C

6. Which statement is NOT true about holism?
   a) Holism requires concentrating on, and thus strengthening, disparate elements.
   b) Holism encompasses all modalities of complementary wellness practices.
   c) Holism seeks overall harmony and balance.
   d) Ambience is a critical factor in creating a holistic experience.

   A

7. What is considered the most healing part of holistic treatment?
   a) spirituality
   c) comfort level
   b) ambience
   d) imparting the sense of touch

   D

8. Why is milk good for the skin?
   a) it absorbs quickly
   c) it has healing properties
   b) it contains lactic acid
   d) it contains vitamin D

   B

9. The common thread in all holistic therapies is:
   a) healing energy
   c) unblocking energy
   b) the power of touch
   d) balancing the elements

   A

10. The effectiveness of a client's treatment is directly proportional to:
    a) the ambience of the treatment room
    b) the amount of touch involved
    c) the amount of time you give them
    d) the overall experience you give them

    D

11. Acupuncture reflects the Chinese belief that when the qi is out of balance:
    a) you require natural therapies
    b) disease and disorder can occur
    c) you cannot transfer positive energy
    d) you can treat the mind but not the body

    B

12. The principles of qi are based on what kind of system?
    a) circulatory
    c) vascular
    b) nervous
    d) energy

    D

13. The goal in achieving qi along the body's 12 energy pathways is to:
    a) enable the body to function at its best
    b) enhance the holistic experience
    c) realize the power of touch
    d) be aware of healing energy

    A

14. Acupressure releases blocked energy along the energy pathways
    by using:
    a) yin and yang   c) meridians
    b) pressure   d) needles

    B
    ___

15. Acupuncture releases blocked energy along the energy path-
    ways by using:
    a) meridians   c) fine needles
    b) pressure   d) aromatherapy

    C
    ___

16. Acupressure and acupuncture are therapies that are considered
    to be:
    a) preventive   c) neither preventive nor healing
    b) healing   d) both preventive and healing

    D
    ___

17. Which of the following does NOT demonstrate the Chinese
    notion of balance and harmony among the universal elements?
    a) dark and light   c) sun and moon
    b) man and woman   d) rest and recuperation

    D
    ___

18. Which is an important aspect of building solid relationships, also
    known as public relations?
    a) thinking individually but not collectively
    b) trying to represent yourself and not the salon or entire profession
    c) setting procedures for addressing customer service and employee
       relations
    d) focusing solely on your business now and thinking about your
       place in the community later

    C
    ___

19. Chinese medicine is based on the belief that life is a coordinated
    practice of:
    a) unblocking energy pathways
    b) harmony between competing forces in the universe
    c) simplicity
    d) enhancing the holistic experience

    B
    ___

20. Essential oils used in aromatherapy can affect this part of the
    brain, which controls emotions:
    a) the limbic system   c) craniosacral system
    b) cranial nerves   d) pituitary gland

    A
    ___

21. The ancient Hindu art of medicine and prolonging life using various methods is:
    a) Ayurvedia
    b) shiodara
    c) Lomi Lomi
    d) Reiki

    A

22. Which of the following statements about Ayurvedia is NOT true?
    a) Ayurvedia means the science of life.
    b) Ayurvedic practices originated in India more than 5,000 years ago.
    c) Ayurvedia is a universal concept of balancing all aspects of medicine.
    d) Ayurvedic treatments involve massage, meditation, breathing, and diet.

    C

23. The Ayurvedic relaxation technique of dripping oil over the forehead is called:
    a) polarity therapy
    b) reflexology
    c) shiatsu
    d) shiodara

    D

24. Which is a type of Japanese massage in which energy flows between two people?
    a) Reiki
    b) Lomi Lomi
    c) craniosacral massage
    d) hydrotherapy

    A

25. Which is a system of movement that balances positive and negative energy?
    a) polarity therapy
    b) the Trager method
    c) Reiki
    d) trigger point myotherapy

    A

26. Who among the following people did not develop a therapeutic treatment?
    a) Dr. William Fitzgerald
    b) Dr. Randolph Stone
    c) Eunice Inghram
    d) Cleopatra

    D

27. Which one of these therapies concentrates on the head and spinal column?
    a) shiatsu
    b) trigger point myotherapy
    c) craniosacral massage
    d) Lomi Lomi

    C

28. Which of the following therapies massages principally the hands and feet?
    a) aromatherapy
    b) Reiki
    c) shiatsu
    d) reflexology

    D

29. Which of the following is NOT true of Lomi Lomi?
    a) It is practiced mostly in Hawaii.
    b) It has spiritual, breathing, and energy components.
    c) It involves large dancelike motions.
    d) It was formerly called zone therapy.

    D

30. What does shiatsu mean?
    a) stress therapy
    b) finger pressure therapy
    c) healing therapy
    d) energy system

    B

31. The Japanese use this word to refer to the motor points of nerves and muscles along the meridians that connect all the organs and systems to one whole.
    a) tsunami
    b) tsubo
    c) sushi
    d) sashimi

    B

32. In the Trager method, the central nervous system releases:
    a) pressure
    b) hormones
    c) stress
    d) doshas

    C

33. Trigger point myotherapy concentrates on relieving what kind of pain?
    a) myofacial
    b) cryofacial
    c) limbic system
    d) thyroidal

    A

34. Which of the following has nothing to do with herbalism?
    a) yoga
    b) vegetarian
    c) macrobiotic
    d) hydrotherapy

    D

Chapter **28**

ADVANCED HOME CARE

1. Clients usually learn about skin care trends through:
   a) word of mouth
   c) media and advertising
   b) their physicians
   d) hygiene classes

   C

2. Dr. Albert Klingman's breakthrough research on Retin-A took place at:
   a) Harvard Medical School
   b) the Food and Drug Administration (FDA)
   c) the National Institutes of Health (NIH)
   d) University of Pennsylvania School of Medicine

   D

3. Deep pore cleansers for home use dissolve oil clogs in follicles with:
   a) resorcinol
   c) alphanucleic acid
   b) beta carotene
   d) beta hydroxy or alpha hydroxy acid

   D

4. The main role of antioxidants is to:
   a) soften sebaceous material
   c) neutralize free radicals
   b) lighten blackheads
   d) accelerate exfoliation

   C

5. Eye cream or gel helps to relieve dark circles by:
   a) tinting the skin around the eye
   b) stimulating microcirculation
   c) suppressing melanin in the skin around the eye
   d) removing dead cell matter

   B

6. A good time to educate clients about new products and product
   choices is:
   a) on the telephone
   b) during exfoliation treatments
   c) during the skin care analysis
   d) while scheduling follow-up appointments

   C

7. During the skin care analysis, you should NOT:
   a) identify specific products
   b) discuss the need for evening hydration
   c) discuss deep pore cleansing
   d) use a magnifying lamp

   A

8. The sheet that outlines step-by-step instructions for the client is
   known as the:
   a) skin care menu   c) the home care treatment form
   b) daily itemization   d) the cosmeceuticals list

   C

9. When selling advanced home care products, it is important to
   emphasize:
   a) ingredients   c) price
   b) client benefits   d) treatment instructions

   B

10. If a product has a high price, you, as an esthetician, should:
    a) not offer the product
    b) try to reduce the price
    c) suggest a payment plan
    d) continue to educate the client about the product

    D

11. A way to enhance your credibility when selling products is to:
    a) attempt to justify higher prices
    b) use the products yourself
    c) sympathize with the client's concerns over high prices
    d) minimize the client's problems

    B

12. When discussing and selling products, an esthetician should
    avoid words like:
    a) improvement   c) correction
    b) enhancement   d) refinement

    C

13. When designing advanced product plans for clients, you should strive for key ingredient synergy, which means the ingredients should all:
    a) be used separately
    b) work together to achieve a single end result
    c) serve to energize the skin
    d) promote improved circulation

    B

14. Which of the following is NOT a characteristic of aging skin?
    a) it experiences a loss of elasticity
    b) it has reduced lipid content
    c) it experiences a loss of pigmentation
    d) its ability to retain water is impaired

    C

15. Intrinsic aging refers to:
    a) environmental skin damage
    b) aging of the skin caused by cumulative illness
    c) aging of the skin caused by dietary habits
    d) the body's normal aging process

    D

16. Cellular components responsible for regenerating collagen and elastin in the skin are:
    a) nuclei   c) neuroblasts
    b) fibroblasts   d) ribosomes

    B

17. Which of the following vitamins does NOT have antioxidative properties?
    a) vitamin B5   c) vitamin E
    b) vitamin C   d) vitamin A

    A

18. Phyto extracts applied to the skin are derived from:
    a) fruits   c) plants
    b) fungi   d) plankton

    C

19. Of the following phyto extracts, which is known to have astringent properties?
    a) ginseng   c) jasmine
    b) pinecone   d) turmeric

    B

20. Of the following lipids, which contains omega-3 fatty acids?
    a) soybean oil
    c) squalane
    b) rice bran oil
    d) orange roughy oil

    D

21. Skin care products meant to enhance circulation impact the:
    a) arteries
    c) capillaries
    b) veins
    d) lymphocytes

    C

22. Which of the following vitamins supports epidermal cell turnover?
    a) vitamin E
    c) vitamin C
    b) vitamin D3
    d) vitamin A

    B

23. Which of the following can improve the lipid barrier?
    a) jojoba oil
    c) hypericum
    b) shea butter
    d) soybean oil

    D

24. Which of the following phyto extracts does NOT have astringent properties?
    a) geranium
    c) horse chestnut
    b) comfrey
    d) guaiazulene

    A

25. Which of the following phyto extracts is a known circulatory stimulant?
    a) lavender
    c) cucumber
    b) hypericum
    d) grape

    C

26. Which of the following ingredients would be most useful for building and retaining a moisture barrier?
    a) elastin
    c) linden
    b) collagen
    d) hyssop

    B

27. Ingredients for problematic or acne skin should emphasize:
    a) emollient properties
    b) lipid content
    c) collagen
    d) antiseptic and antimicrobial properties

    D

28. Which of the following exfoliants is NOT an alpha hydroxy acid?
    a) malic acid
    c) lactic acid
    b) salicylic acid
    d) glycolic acid

    B

29. For treating problematic skin, the botanical aloe vera is utilized
    for this property:
    a) antiseptic   c) exfoliative
    b) soothing   d) comedogenic

30. Of the ingredients categorized as "special agents" for treating
    problematic skin, which has the ability to enhance cell metabolism?
    a) glycerin   c) glycoproteins
    b) colloidal sulfur   d) yeast beta-glucans

Chapter 29

METHODS OF HAIR REMOVAL

1. How much hair you have is determined by:
   - a) sweat glands
   - b) genetics
   - c) the nervous system
   - d) anxiety levels

   B

2. Hair is formed from a hard protein called:
   - a) keratin
   - b) collagen
   - c) carotene
   - d) cartilage

   A

3. Which of the following statements is false?
   - a) A hair follicle is a mass of epidermis extending down into the dermis.
   - b) The follicle swells at the base to form a hair bulb.
   - c) All follicles contain a hair shaft.
   - d) Follicles grow all over the body.

   C

4. The base of the follicle contains an oval-shaped cavity filled with tissue called:
   - a) sebaceous gland
   - b) pilosebaceous
   - c) dermal papilla
   - d) arrector pili

   C

5. Which is the outer layer of the hair shaft?
   - a) medulla
   - b) cuticle
   - c) cortex
   - d) dermal papilla

   B

6. Which is the innermost layer of the hair shaft?
   - a) cuticle
   - b) cortex
   - c) medulla
   - d) epidermis

   C

cortex medulla cortex — cuticle

7. Which is the in-between layer of the hair shaft?
   a) medulla   c) keratin
   b) cortex   d) cuticle

   B ?

8. Where are hair color changes made?
   a) cortex   c) medulla
   b) hair bulb   d) cuticle

   A

9. Which of the following statements is false?
   a) The hair bulb nourishes the growing basal part of the hair.
   b) Pilosebaceous follicles contain both the sebaceous appendage and hair shaft.
   c) The hair follicle surrounds the lower part of the hair shaft.
   d) The root is the part of the hair that lies just outside the follicle.

   D

10. What is the function of the sebaceous glands?
    a) lubricate the skin and hair
    b) stimulate the follicles
    c) contain the blood vessels and cells necessary for hair growth
    d) allow hair to reach the surface of the skin

    A

11. Which is NOT needed for strong, healthy hair?
    a) vitamins   c) nutrients
    b) minerals   d) anagen

    D

12. The face contains approximately how many follicles per square inch?
    a) 3,200   c) 320
    b) 32,000   d) 320,000

    A

13. How is new hair formed?
    a) The hair bulb brings nutrients to the blood vessels to form new hair.
    b) Blood vessels bring nutrients to the base of the hair bulb, causing it to grow.
    c) Sebaceous glands lubricate the hair and stimulate the follicles.
    d) Nutrients in the blood stimulate keratinocytes.

    B

14. When does hair formation begin?
    a) before birth   c) between birth and 3 months
    b) just after birth   d) after age 1

    A

15. The hair on a fetus is called:
    a) hypertrichosis
    b) vellus hair
    c) lanugo
    d) lanolin

    C

16. Which of the following hair characteristics is NOT determined before birth?
    a) secretion activity
    b) depth of the hair shaft
    c) color
    d) how quickly it grows

    D

17. The growth stage of hair is known as:
    a) telogen
    b) vellus
    c) catagen
    d) anagen

    D

18. Vellus hair is most likely to be found on the:
    a) top of the head
    b) cheeks
    c) eyebrows
    d) pubic region

    B

19. Persistently dull, lifeless hair is often a sign of:
    a) trichinosis
    b) poor health
    c) poor hygiene
    d) a dysfunctional hair growth cycle

    B

20. In warm climates, hair tends to:
    a) grow more slowly
    b) lose its luster
    c) grow more rapidly
    d) fall out more quickly

    C

21. The term hirsutism refers to:
    a) hair growth in regions where hair does not normally grow
    b) excessive hair growth on the face, arms, and legs
    c) excessively curly hair
    d) hair that is excessively coarse in texture

    B

22. Hirsutism is a condition that most often affects:
    a) women
    b) men
    c) children
    d) Hispanics

    A

23. Female hirsutism usually indicates:
    a) insufficient levels of androgens
    b) an overabundance of hair follicles
    c) an overabundance of sebaceous glands
    d) excessive levels of androgens

    D

24. Which one of the following is NOT a cause of female hirsutism?
    a) pregnancy
    c) vitamin deficiency
    b) age
    d) menopause

    B

25. Which of the following statements is NOT true?
    a) Hair filters out dust and other airborne particles.
    b) Hair protects the body from environmental elements.
    c) Hair allows secretions to move up and out onto the skin's surface.
    d) Some people have no body hair due to their geographic location.

    D

26. Hair removal tends to be easier but the skin is more sensitive in people who have what color hair?
    a) black
    c) brown
    b) red and blond
    d) auburn

    B

27. How did people acquire mixed traits of hair color and thickness?
    a) advances in hair dye and removal systems
    b) environmental changes due to weather and geography
    c) the migration of cultures from region to region
    d) ultraviolet rays

    C

28. Skin and hair tend to be thicker and darker in people who live:
    a) closer to the equator
    c) near the South Pole
    b) near the North Pole
    d) in the Western part of
    the world

    A

29. Which of the following statements is false?
    a) Individuals with olive skin tones tend to have pigmentation problems.
    b) Australians tend to have black, coarse, curly hair.
    c) Central and South American cultures have darker, more noticeable hair.
    d) Native Americans tend toward thick hair and roots that are close to the surface.

    D

30. Hair can only be permanently removed with:
    a) the destruction of the papilla
    b) epilation
    c) breaking contact between the bulb and the papilla
    d) chemical depilation

    A

31. Barbae folliculitis means:
    a) infected hair follicle
    c) ingrown hair
    b) immature hair follicle
    d) the papilla is destroyed

    C

32. Where should you patch test a chemical depilatory?
    a) upper thigh   c) palm of your hand
    b) inside of the arm   d) sole of your foot   *B*

33. A melting point is the temperature at which a substance:
    a) hardens   c) liquefies
    b) drips   d) becomes clear   *C*

34. Which of the following statements about hair removal
    techniques is FALSE?
    a) Wax should adhere to the hair as close to the skin as possible.
    b) Many estheticians prefer roll-on wax because it is sanitary.
    c) Threading uses a sewing needle to insert wax in hard-to-reach areas.
    d) Sugaring is a water-soluble method dating back to the Egyptians.   *C*

35. Which hair removal method is NOT considered permanent?
    a) sugaring   c) laser
    b) electrolysis   d) photo light   *A*

36. Which is NOT a type of electrolysis?
    a) galvanic   c) thermolysis
    b) electrodialysis   d) blend   *B*

37. Which of the following statements is false?
    a) Light colors absorb more light.
    b) A laser produces colored light.
    c) A laser is a direct beam of light.
    d) Light is energy.   *A*

38. Laser light passes harmlessly through the skin and targets only
    the what?
    a) white blood cell
    b) hemoglobin of the red blood cell
    c) diode
    d) saline moisture inside the follicle   *B*

39. When selecting a waxing table, it is important to make sure the
    table is:
    a) light in color
    b) height-adjustable
    c) aluminum
    d) rounded on the corners to minimize injury   *B*

40. Waxing heaters should:
    a) be high-capacity
    b) be kerosene-powered
    c) carry a warranty
    d) be made in the USA

    C

41. A waxing room should have a covered waste can that is:
    a) plastic
    b) metal
    c) sterile
    d) foot-operated

    D

42. Epilation tools and supplies must be replenished:
    a) weekly
    b) monthly
    c) hourly
    d) daily

    D

43. Professional tweezers should be made of:
    a) aircraft aluminum
    b) stainless steel
    c) galvanized steel
    d) zinc-plated steel

    B

44. When purchasing tweezers, a good rule of thumb is:
    a) buyer beware
    b) the largest point size is the best point size
    c) buy the best you can afford
    d) always choose the most expensive offering

    C

45. A pointed-tip tweezer is well suited for:
    a) general tweezing
    b) removing ingrown hair
    c) removing blonde hair
    d) removing curly hair

    B

46. For spreading thin coats of wax on large areas, the best choice is:
    a) cotton pads
    b) cotton swabs
    c) wooden sticks
    d) a stainless steel spatula

    D

47. Stainless steel instruments should be sanitized either in solution or with:
    a) microwaves
    b) steam
    c) an autoclave
    d) x-rays

    C

48. Prior to waxing, it is a good idea to apply a solution that:
    a) depigments the skin
    b) degreases the skin
    c) shrinks the follicles
    d) roughens the skin

    B

49. Tea tree oil may be added to post-waxing solutions to help:
    a) calm the skin   c) protect the skin from sun exposure
    b) contract the follicles   d) dissolve any remaining hair   *A*

50. Client health forms must be completed:
    a) only by clients undergoing electrolysis
    b) during epilation as part of a monitoring process
    c) before epilation
    d) after epilation   *C*

51. The main purpose of the client health form is to:
    a) provide the client's social security number
    b) point out potential contraindications to treatment
    c) provide the client's billing information
    d) serve as a liability waiver   *B*

52. Clients taking blood thinners such as Coumadin:
    a) can never undergo waxing
    b) should stop their medication 48 hours prior to waxing
    c) can undergo waxing only if their physician authorizes the procedure
    d) are particularly good candidates for waxing   *C*

53. Waxing strips that do NOT shed or stretch are made of:
    a) cotton   c) papyrus
    b) muslin   d) pellon   *D*

54. When waxing, an esthetician should wear gloves made of:
    a) latex   c) leather
    b) vinyl   d) cotton   *B*

55. Blood-stained gauze should be:
    a) treated like any other waste   c) rinsed and reused
    b) burned   d) placed in a hazardous
                                     waste container   *D*

56. Talcum powder should NOT be used after waxing because:
    a) it is messy
    b) it may cause an allergic reaction
    c) it is too fragrant
    d) it adds unnecessary cost to the procedure   *B*

57. When working with hard wax, the wax should be applied:
    a) in a circular motion
    b) in a figure-eight pattern
    c) to the thickness of a dime
    d) using a 4" X 4" cotton gauze pad

    B

58. When removing strip wax it is important to pull the strips off:
    a) very slowly and gently
    b) in the same direction as the hair growth
    c) multiple times in halting motions
    d) in the opposite direction of the hair growth

    D

Chapter *30*

WAXING PROCEDURES

1. The most commonly requested wax service is:
   a) eyebrow arching
   b) waxing the ear
   c) waxing the upper torso
   d) waxing the leg

   A

2. The strip wax method is used for:
   a) waxing the lip
   b) waxing the cheek
   c) brow waxing
   d) waxing the chin

   C

3. Which of the following behaviors demonstrates a bad work ethic?
   a) attending a seminar on new techniques
   b) being late or absent from work
   c) accepting criticism
   d) soliciting your boss' input on ways to improve a treatment

   B

4. The space between the eyes should be equal to:
   a) the width of one eye
   b) the width of two eyes
   c) the width of the nose
   d) the width of the mouth

   A

5. After facial services, the most popular hair removal service is waxing the:
   a) shoulders and back
   b) underarm
   c) hands
   d) leg

   D

6. About how long does leg waxing last?
   a) 1 to 2 weeks
   b) 2 to 3 weeks
   c) 4 to 6 weeks
   d) 6 to 7 weeks

   C

7. Why is shaving an unsatisfactory way to remove hair from the upper torso?
   a) Shaving causes ingrown hairs to develop.
   b) Shaving causes the hair to grow back quickly.
   c) Shaving costs too much.
   d) Shaving is painful.

   B

8. What is the appropriate method of removing hair inside the ear cavity?
   a) waxing
   b) clipping with cuticle scissors
   c) pulling out the hair with tweezers
   d) applying depilatory cream

   B

9. What is another word for "hair removal"?
   a) epilation
   b) epidural
   c) appellation
   d) epinephrine

   A

10. What is the proper way of removing wax?
    a) Pull the wax off in the direction of hair growth.
    b) Pull the wax off against the direction of hair growth.
    c) Pull the wax from both ends until it meets in the middle.
    d) Dissolve the wax gently with warm water.

    B

11. What can be used to soothe irritated areas of the skin?
    a) rubbing alcohol
    b) baby oil
    c) cool tea bags
    d) witch hazel

    C

12. When would you recommend electrolysis?
    a) for removal of deep-rooted, coarse facial hair
    b) for removal of nasal hair
    c) for removal of hair in the ear
    d) I would never recommend electrolysis.

    A

13. Which of the following methods of removing ingrown hairs is NOT allowed in some states?
    a) waxing
    b) use of a lancet
    c) use of a tweezer
    d) electrolysis

    B

14. How would you schedule a client with a major ingrown hair problem?
    a) No special scheduling is needed.
    b) extra 30-minute appointment
    c) extra one-hour appointment
    d) two 30-minute sessions at least two days apart

    B

15. When epilating calves, the client should:
     a) sit however she is comfortable   c) lie on her stomach
     b) lie on her back   d) sit with her feet slightly
                                               elevated   *C*

16. The calves are divided into:
     a) three sections: inner, outer, middle
     b) four sections: top, middle, bottom, ankle
     c) three sections: inner, outer, front
     d) two sections: inner and outer   *A*

17. For a bikini line service:
     a) Include upper leg hair.
     b) Ask the client to specify the exact area for hair removal.
     c) Ask the client to wear her bathing suit during the procedure.
     d) Always recommend electrolysis instead of waxing.   *B*

18. To help prevent ingrown hairs, suggest that the client:
     a) use a loofa sponge
     b) apply a cool tea bag on the skin
     c) ingrown hairs cannot be prevented
     d) soak for a half-hour in a bath at least 24 hours before treatment *A*

19. Arm hair epilation presents a special challenge because:
     a) The arm is a sensitive area.
     b) Arm hair tends to grow in different directions.
     c) Full removal of arm hair requires several appointments.
     d) Arm hair tends to be deep-rooted.   *B*

20. Which of the following items should you use to check your work
     after a waxing procedure?
     a) camera   c) magnifying lamp
     b) microscope   d) mirror   *C*

21. Following a waxing procedure, for how many hours should the
     client refrain from exposing the waxed area to sun or a tanning
     bed?
     a) 24 hours   c) 48 hours
     b) 36 hours   d) 72 hours   *C*

22. What is a muslin strip used for?
    a) soothing irritated areas of the skin
    b) cleaning areas of the skin
    c) treating ingrown hairs
    d) removing hair

    D

23. What is the correct way to hold a spatula when waxing the shoulder area?
    a) facing up
    b) facing down
    c) at an angle
    d) You should not use a spatula during waxing.

    C

24. Shaving the underarm can cause:
    a) ingrown hairs
    b) growth of bacteria
    c) development of deep-rooted hair
    d) permanent loss of hair

    A

25. What is the correct way of discarding hard wax?
    a) Recycle it.
    b) Discard it with the regular trash.
    c) Burn it.
    d) Discard it in a hazardous waste container.

    D

26. Which of the following areas has hair that typically grows in several directions?
    a) chin   c) underarm
    b) upper lip   d) cheek

    C

27. When waxing only the shoulder area, how should the client be positioned?
    a) The client lies face up.
    b) The client lies on his or her side.
    c) The client may sit or lie face down on the table.
    d) The client stands.

    C

28. When waxing the entire back, how should the client be positioned?
    a) The client lies on his or her side.
    b) The client stands.
    c) The client lies face up.
    d) The client lies face down.

    D

29. When waxing the entire back, section the back into:
    a) two parts   c) four parts
    b) three parts   d) five parts

    C

30. What should you do if a drop of wax accidentally falls into your client's eyelashes?
    a) ask the client to close eyes gently, then apply petroleum jelly
    b) wash with cool water
    c) ask the client to squeeze eyes tight, then apply witch hazel
    d) ignore it

    A

31. Which of the following steps should you take before applying wax to the client's skin?
    a) stir the wax
    b) test the temperature of the wax
    c) taste the wax
    d) add water to the wax

    B

32. When brow waxing, apply a thin coat of wax:
    a) from the outside to the inside of the orbital bone with one swipe
    b) from the inside to the outside of the orbital bone with one swipe
    c) from the inside to the outside of the orbital bone with several swipes
    d) on the outside of the orbital bone

    B

33. For eyebrow shaping, which of the following tools can be used to mark your points?
    a) orangewood stick   c) pen
    b) muslin strip   d) crayon

    A

34. What is a common result of applying too much pressure when applying a muslin strip?
    a) bleeding   c) numbness
    b) bruising   d) acne

    B

35. How do you find the arch of the eyebrow?
    a) Ask your client to show you where it is.
    b) Line up the pencil along the outside edge of the iris.
    c) Use a ruler to measure.
    d) You should avoid the arch area.

    B

36. What is the step after examining the brow and determining the shape?
    a) brush the brows into a smooth line
    b) remove excess hairs
    c) hand the client a mirror
    d) rinse the area thoroughly

    _A_

37. Why do you hand the client a mirror after brushing the brows into a smooth line?
    a) to allow the client to evaluate the work you have already done
    b) to discuss exactly where hair will be removed
    c) to allow the client to evaluate the work as you do it
    d) all of the above are correct

    _B_

38. What should you do with brows over close-set eyes?
    a) remove the brow hairs just beyond the inner corner of the eye
    b) remove the brow hairs just beyond the outer corner of the eye
    c) extend the brows to equal the distance between the eyes
    d) none of the above are correct

    _A_

39. Why do you trim any especially long brow hairs before brow waxing?
    a) a few less hairs make all the difference when shaping
    b) helps the wax adhere
    c) allows you to remove the hair more easily and comfortably
    d) all of the above are correct

    _D_

40. When waxing the underarm, why do you place a towel over the client's chest?
    a) for privacy
    b) for warmth
    c) for perspiration
    d) to protect the chest from spills or drips

    _D_

41. What is the best way to determine the direction of hair growth on the arm?
    a) feel the skin with your hand
    b) comb the hair
    c) pour water onto the hair
    d) ask the client to determine the direction

    _A_

42. What is the final step in the procedure for waxing the underarm?
    a) Trim any remaining hairs with scissors.
    b) Wipe the area, making sure that no wax residue is left.
    c) Remove the client's head protection.
    d) Pour a few drops of postwax soothing solution on the area.

    C

43. Why should you hold the client's upper leg taught during bikini waxing?
    a) It prevents the leg from falling asleep.
    b) It prevents skin tears and bruising.
    c) It is comfortable for the client.
    d) It prevents ingrown hairs.

    B

44. Before applying the wax to an area, you need to make sure that:
    a) the area is wet
    b) the area is warm
    c) the area is dry
    d) the area is covered with petroleum jelly

    C

45. What is the main reason for reviewing the client history form before performing a procedure?
    a) to make sure there are no contraindications
    b) to make sure the client can pay for the service
    c) to verify that the client is old enough to receive the service
    d) Reviewing the client history form is not necessary.

    A

46. Which of the following steps is part of setting up a waxing procedure area?
    a) turn on loud music
    b) dim the lights
    c) prepare the waxing table or bed with fresh paper
    d) no preparation is needed

    C

47. Which of the following procedures is considered controversial?
    a) electrolysis
    b) Brazilian bikini waxing
    c) ingrown hair service
    d) waxing the ear

    B

48. For the hard wax method, how much wax should you apply to the area?
    a) Apply the wax to the thickness of a dime.
    b) Apply the wax to the thickness of a quarter.
    c) Apply the wax to the thickness of a nickel.
    d) Apply the wax to the thickness of your thumb.

    C

Chapter **31**

COLOR THEORY, FACIAL FEATURES, AND SETUP

1. In the 1980s, color analysis was based upon:
   a) body analysis
   b) seasons
   c) natural beauty
   d) overall look

   B

2. Over the past ten years makeup formulas were transformed to include:
   a) vitamins and minerals
   b) sunscreen
   c) botanical extracts
   d) all of the above are correct

   D

3. Another name for color is:
   a) tint
   b) value
   c) hue
   d) shade

   C

4. Red, yellow, and blue are called:
   a) secondary colors
   b) primary colors
   c) tertiary colors
   d) complementary colors

   B

5. Every color or hue is developed from:
   a) complementary colors
   b) shade of a color
   c) intermediate colors
   d) primary colors

   D

6. One primary and one secondary color opposite each other on the color wheel are called:
   a) complementary colors
   b) tertiary colors
   c) secondary colors
   d) primary colors

   A

7. When black is added to a color, we are creating:
   a) tint
   b) intensity
   c) shade
   d) value

   C

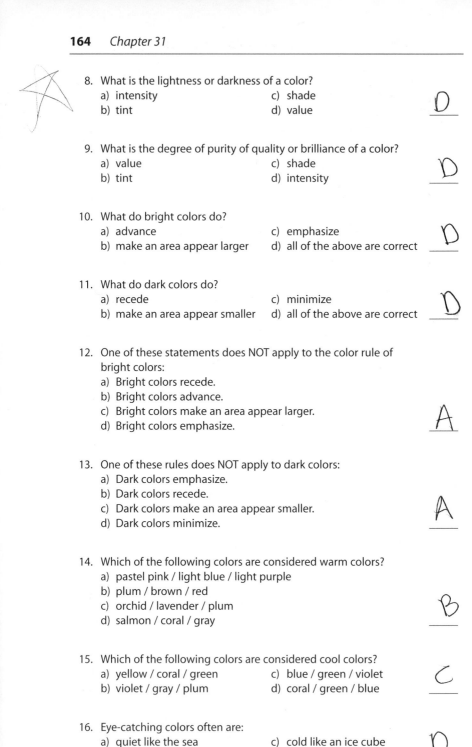

8. What is the lightness or darkness of a color?
   a) intensity   c) shade
   b) tint   d) value

   D

9. What is the degree of purity of quality or brilliance of a color?
   a) value   c) shade
   b) tint   d) intensity

   D

10. What do bright colors do?
    a) advance   c) emphasize
    b) make an area appear larger   d) all of the above are correct

    D

11. What do dark colors do?
    a) recede   c) minimize
    b) make an area appear smaller   d) all of the above are correct

    D

12. One of these statements does NOT apply to the color rule of bright colors:
    a) Bright colors recede.
    b) Bright colors advance.
    c) Bright colors make an area appear larger.
    d) Bright colors emphasize.

    A

13. One of these rules does NOT apply to dark colors:
    a) Dark colors emphasize.
    b) Dark colors recede.
    c) Dark colors make an area appear smaller.
    d) Dark colors minimize.

    A

14. Which of the following colors are considered warm colors?
    a) pastel pink / light blue / light purple
    b) plum / brown / red
    c) orchid / lavender / plum
    d) salmon / coral / gray

    B

15. Which of the following colors are considered cool colors?
    a) yellow / coral / green   c) blue / green / violet
    b) violet / gray / plum   d) coral / green / blue

    C

16. Eye-catching colors often are:
    a) quiet like the sea   c) cold like an ice cube
    b) shaded like a mountain   d) used in advertising

    D

17. Colors that are bright and attention-getting remind us of summer or excitement. They are:
    a) quiet like the sea   c) cool colors
    b) shaded like a mountain   d) warm colors

    D

18. What colors promote a more relaxed and quiet state of mind?
    a) bright colors   c) warm colors
    b) attention-getting colors   d) cool colors

    D

19. Which of these colors combines well with other colors?
    a) white   c) black
    b) gray   d) all of the above are correct

    D

20. Which of these colors is NOT neutral?
    a) black   c) white
    b) brown   d) gray

    B

21. What needs to be determined for a makeup profiling by an image consultant?
    a) skin type   c) hair color / eye color / skin tone
    b) body type   d) all of the above are correct

    D

22. What skin tone do tanned Caucasians have?
    a) beige   c) olive
    b) dark   d) ivory

    C

23. What skin tone do medium Caucasians have?
    a) fair   c) beige
    b) deep   d) olive

    C

24. What skin undertone do light Asians have?
    a) creamy   c) yellow
    b) brown/yellow   d) orange/red

    A

25. What are the undertones of a dark Hispanic skin?
    a) gold/yellow   c) slightly pink
    b) yellow   d) brown/yellow

    D

26. Pink or yellow skin undertones are seen in which ethnic group?
    a) tanned Caucasians   c) medium Caucasians
    b) dark Hispanics   d) light Caucasians

    C

27. Olive or warm skin tones are seen in which ethnic group?
    a) medium Hispanic   c) medium Caucasians
    b) light Asians   d) very black

    A

28. What is the standard face shape which all other shapes are measured by?
    a) round   c) oval
    b) triangle   d) heart

    C

29. What face shape is long and narrow, with an overly long angular chin and a big forehead?
    a) inverted triangle   c) rectangular
    b) heart   d) diamond

    C

30. Which of the following face shapes has an angular jawline and not particularly prominent cheekbones?
    a) square   c) triangle
    b) rectangular   d) heart

    A

31. Which face shape is widest at the cheekbone area, and is usually not much longer than its width?
    a) square   c) diamond
    b) oval   d) round

    D

32. What is the widest part of a triangular face?
    a) the temples   c) the cheekbones
    b) the jawline   d) the forehead

    B

33. How is the face divided lengthwise?
    a) horizontally into 5 divisions   c) lengthwise into 5 divisions
    b) vertically into 3 divisions   d) horizontally into 3 divisions

    D

34. What determines the width of the face?
    a) the width of the mouth
    b) the width of the nose
    c) the space between the eyebrows and the base of the nose
    d) the space between the eyes

    D

35. Application of color on the cheeks should start from:
    a) the lip area   c) the middle of the iris
    b) the nostrils   d) one to two finger widths
                                 from the nostrils

    D

36. What serves as the basis of makeup?
    a) patterns and colors   c) highlighting
    b) face shapes and proportions d) shadowing

    B

37. Where should eyebrows start?
    a) at the inner edge of the eye   c) the middle of the nostrils
    b) at the outer edge of the eye   d) at the outer edge of the iris

    A

38. What eyebrow shape tends to make eyes look smaller?
    a) Asian   c) arched
    b) straight d) curved

    B

39. What eyebrow shape tends to give the face a surprised look?
    a) straight c) arched
    b) Asian   d) curved

    C

40. Which brows tend to be straight or slightly curved, with hair growing in a downward direction?
    a) arched   c) curved
    b) straight d) Asian

    D

41. What gives the eyes a vacant or empty expression?
    a) brows that grow downward
    b) brows that have no curves
    c) angled lines above the natural brow bone
    d) an extreme curve to the brow

    D

42. What are the divisions of the eye?
    a) the eyelid   c) the brow bone
    b) the depth area d) all of the above are correct

    D

43. What is the measurement of a well-proportioned eye area from the base of the lashes to the eyebrow?
    a) two-thirds and one-third c) one-third and two-thirds
    b) the width of one eye   d) half and half

    C

44. Well-shaped eyes have the width of:
    a) one eye between them   c) one eyebrow between them
    b) one mouth between them   d) a nostril between them

    A

45. What is one of the correction techniques for hidden eyelids?
    a) applying dark shadow on the crease
    b) applying mascara only at the outer corners of the eyes
    c) highlighting the brow bone
    d) applying shadow at the outer corners of the lower lids

    C

46. What is one of the correction techniques for deep-set eyes?
    a) applying mascara upward and outward
    b) using soft color
    c) applying highlight to the brow bone
    d) lining inside the eyes

    B

47. To offset the droop of the eye it is necessary to give the appearance of a lift by:
    a) using soft colors
    b) using dark shadow
    c) lining the inside of the eyes
    d) applying highlight under the arch

    D

48. When the hooded area is shadowed and the area below it is highlighted, what nose shape are we trying to bring to balance with the face?
    a) a long nose
    b) a hooked nose
    c) a short nose
    d) a broad nose

    B

49. When we shadow the base and the tip of the nose, what nose shape we are trying to balance?
    a) a short nose
    b) a crooked nose
    c) a broad nose
    d) a long nose

    D

50. Lining the lower lip and filling in with lip color to create balance between the lower and upper lip is a corrective technique for what lip shape?
    a) thin upper and lower lip
    b) uneven lips
    c) small mouth and lips
    d) thin lower lip

    D

51. For what lip shape do we line the lips to build the corners of the mouth?
    a) cupid bow upper lip
    b) drooping corners
    c) uneven lips
    d) straight upper lip

    B

52. How many foundation types are there?
    a) tinted moisturizers and creams
    b) four types
    c) creams and liquids
    d) two types in a combination

    B

53. Which one of these is NOT a foundation?
    a) cream
    b) tinted moisturizer
    c) concealer
    d) mineral powder

    C

54. The foundation should match:
    a) the neck
    b) the cheeks
    c) the hand
    d) the forehead

    B

55. Which of the following have the smallest number of skin variations in color tones?
    a) Asian skin
    b) Hispanic skin
    c) Caucasian skin
    d) black skin

    C

56. Applying a darker foundation from below the cheekbones and along the jaw line and blending into the neck is contouring this face type:
    a) narrow face
    b) wide jaw
    c) long, heavy chin
    d) double chin

    B

57. The purpose of powders is:
    a) to pack the skin
    b) to set foundation
    c) to color-correct a foundation
    d) all of the above are correct

    D

58. What is used to even out eye area and make the eye shadow stick or keep from creasing?
    a) eyebrow pencil
    b) eyeliner pencil
    c) eye shadow base
    d) eye shadow

    C

59. What is used to outline, fill in, highlight, or diminish some imperfections?
    a) eyeliner pencil
    b) lip pencil
    c) eyebrow pencil
    d) all of the above are correct

    D

60. Which brush is designed to apply eye shadow to the eye area from the lashes to the brow?
    a) eyeliner brush
    b) fluff brush
    c) angled, stiff brush
    d) fan brush

    B

61. What brush is used to spread colors onto cheeks to give the face a rosy glow?
    a) powder brush
    b) fan brush
    c) lip brush
    d) blush brush

    D

62. Which of the following are disposable tools?
    a) tweezers
    b) makeup palettes
    c) mascara wands and lip brushes
    d) eyelash curlers

63. What lighting is the most preferable in a makeup room?
    a) cool and warm light
    b) cool fluorescent light
    c) warm light
    d) daylight

Chapter *32*

MAKEUP APPLICATIONS

1. Which of the following does NOT belong in a makeup work area setup?
   a) bar stool
   b) antique furniture
   c) makeup workstation
   d) used tools

   D

2. Which one of these standard consultation forms lists the colors, products, and accessories used during the makeup session?
   a) makeup profile
   b) face makeup chart
   c) confidential makeup questionnaire
   d) skin analysis form

   B

3. Which one of these standard forms for a makeup consultation is filled out as each step of the makeup session is completed?
   a) makeup profile
   b) confidential makeup questionnaire
   c) makeup chart
   d) skin analysis form

   A

4. Which one of these forms is to be completed by the client upon arrival?
   a) makeup profile
   b) confidential makeup questionnaire
   c) makeup chart
   d) skin analysis form

   B

5. What is the purpose of the basic makeup consultation?
   a) to develop a makeup look
   b) to complete confidential makeup profile
   c) tidy makeup area
   d) to set up more appointments

   A

6. Which of the following is part of client preparation?
   a) place a clean makeup drape on the chair
   b) cleanse the lips
   c) choose an appropriate foundation
   d) greet the client and escort her to makeup area

   D

7. Which one of these steps should be done first, before applying makeup?
   a) applying foundation   c) applying loose powder
   b) applying toner   d) applying concealer

   B

8. Which one of the following is the actual cleansing procedure?
   a) cleanse the eyes with a downward stroke
   b) cleanse the lips with an outer to inner movement
   c) remove makeup and debris from the face
   d) cleanse the face of extra mascara

   C

9. Foundation is applied by using:
   a) the fingers   c) a brush
   b) cotton balls   d) a sponge

   D

10. Where is a medium brown color eye shadow applied?
    a) in the crease of the eye   c) from brow to lashes
    b) from lashes to brow bone   d) over the lid again

    A

11. For what part of makeup application do you choose a color that enhances the blood tone?
    a) loose powder   c) concealer
    b) foundation   d) lipstick

    D

12. Which one of the following should complement blush and eye shadow colors?
    a) foundation   c) mascara color
    b) eye pencil   d) lipstick

    D

13. What is one of the drawbacks of custom blended collections?
    a) look-alike-products   c) products for specific purposes
    b) a major initial investment d) inventory surpluses

    B

14. What is one of the benefits of private label products?
    a) large variety of color choices   c) limited products and colors
    b) small or large color ranges   d) great for market uniqueness

    A

15. What line is most cost effective to begin?
    a) specialty lines   c) branded line
    b) private label   d) custom blended

    B

16. Which of these lines is a miscellaneous makeup line?
    a) custom blended   c) branded line
    b) private label   d) specialty lines

    D

17. For what occasion would you use more colorful products?
    a) wedding   c) fantasy
    b) corrective   d) camouflage

    C

18. Which of the following is considered a specialty makeup?
    a) corrective   c) camouflage
    b) wedding   d) all of the above

    D

19. What is paramedical makeup?
    a) 4th of July parade   c) corrective
    b) a mother returning to work   d) camouflage

    D

20. Camouflage makeup is for:
    a) men in a bridal party   c) Halloween
    b) skin disfigurement   d) minor imperfections

    B

21. How can the esthetician/makeup artist keep up with new make-up trends?
    a) watch local music TV stations
    b) subscribe to skin care and makeup journals
    c) attend beauty shows and conventions
    d) all of the above are correct

    D

22. Where in the salon would you place makeup?
    a) in a small area   c) out of the way
    b) in the center   d) in the facial treatment room

    B

Chapter *33*

THE VALUE OF BODY SERVICES

1. Approximately what percentage of the American population turned 50 in the year 2000?
    - a) 25%
    - b) 40%
    - c) 50%
    - d) 60%

    C
    _____

2. Until recently, body treatments were second in importance to what aspect of the esthetics business?
    - a) facial treatments
    - b) electrolysis
    - c) botox treatments
    - d) Body treatments are not an important aspect of the esthetics business.

    A
    _____

3. Which of the following factors does NOT explain the spa boom in the United States?
    - a) aging population
    - b) renewed interest in preventive medicine and wellness
    - c) problems with medical care and insurance programs
    - d) egomania

    D
    _____

4. Which of the following steps is NOT one of the three basic steps performed in spa body treatments?
    - a) cleansing and exfoliation
    - b) skin treatment
    - c) shaving
    - d) body stimulation

    C
    _____

5. What aspect of spa body treatments has changed dramatically in recent years?
   a) technology
   b) state laws
   c) procedures
   d) There have been no dramatic changes in spa body treatments in recent years.

   A
   ___

6. Which of the following is NOT a type of facial?
   a) back facial   c) full body facial
   b) scalp facial   d) foot facial

   D
   ___

7. Who can you call to determine who is allowed to perform body treatments and massage treatments in your state?
   a) health department   c) any health club
   b) recreation department d) a hospital

   A
   ___

8. In some areas of the United States, massage and body treatments come under the authority of:
   a) the Salvation Army   c) the local chamber of commerce
   b) the Red Cross   d) the local vice squad

   D
   ___

9. Why do you not have to worry about pigmentation and wrinkling on the hidden parts of the body?
   a) These parts should not be treated because they are too private.
   b) Clothing usually protects these areas from ultraviolet rays.
   c) These areas are overly sensitive and should be avoided.
   d) Some state licensing boards only allow licensed medical professionals to treat these areas.

   B
   ___

10. In some states, who are the only ones who can perform body treatments?
    a) licensed massage therapists   c) doctors
    b) fitness instructors   d) physical therapists

    A
    ___

11. What is the most appropriate time to discuss the issue of privacy with your client?
    a) before the service
    b) during the service
    c) after the service
    d) Privacy is not an issue for most clients.

    A
    ___

12. Today, what is probably the most important issue in the spa?
    a) privacy
    b) expenses
    c) sanitation
    d) equal treatment of men and women

    C

13. What should be visible in all treatment areas of the spa?
    a) towels
    b) disinfectants
    c) exit signs
    d) first aid kit

    B

14. The health history on the intake form is used for what purpose?
    a) diagnosing disorders
    b) treating disorders
    c) determining the appropriate treatment
    d) The health history is not important.

    C

15. Which of the following is NOT one of the three common elements in the approaches to body and facial treatments?
    a) cleansing and exfoliation
    b) skin treatment
    c) meditation
    d) metabolic stimulation

    C

16. What is the purpose of exfoliation?
    a) prepares the body for a more intensive treatment
    b) soothes irritated areas of the skin
    c) removes wrinkles
    d) moisturizes the skin

    A

17. Which of the following is NOT a type of treatment used for metabolic stimulation?
    a) stimulating mask
    b) cellulite treatment
    c) remineralization
    d) exfoliation

    D

18. What is layering?
    a) scheduling appointments throughout the day
    b) a form of hydrotherapy
    c) mixing and matching treatments
    d) a mud treatment

    C

19. What is hydrotherapy?
    a) physical therapy using hydrogen gas
    b) physical therapy using water
    c) physical therapy using mechanical instruments
    d) physical therapy using salt

    B

20. What is posttreatment stabilization?
    a) relaxing after a stimulating treatment
    b) evaluating the treatment
    c) aromatherapy
    d) exercising to improve circulation

    A

21. When the client is in the prone position, he or she is:
    a) lying face up   c) standing up
    b) lying face down   d) kneeling

    B

22. When the client is in the supine position, he or she is:
    a) kneeling   c) standing up
    b) lying face down   d) lying face up

    D

23. Which of the following is NOT one of the three basic steps performed in most body treatments?
    a) table preparation   c) aromatherapy
    b) client positioning   d) applying product

    C

24. How should clients be positioned for the application of slippery products such as a mud or seaweed wrap?
    a) prone position   c) lying on his or her side
    b) supine position   d) standing up

    B

25. How is the client positioned at the beginning of a body scrub?
    a) face up   c) standing up
    b) face down   d) kneeling down

    B

26. For gommage, salt glow, or body scrub, how is the product applied?
    a) in a back-and-forth motion
    b) in a circular motion
    c) in a sweeping motion
    d) varies according to the client's needs

    B

27. What is the purpose of a granular scrub?
    a) moisturizes the skin   c) removes ingrown hairs
    b) relieves muscle tension   d) removes dead skin cells

    D

28. What is the most common form of skin care gommage products?
    a) liquid   c) cream
    b) powder   d) gel

    C

29. Which of the following is used for dry brushing?
    a) a loofah mitt   c) a sponge
    b) a towel   d) a toothbrush

    A

30. Which of the following is NOT an appropriate approach to marketing your spa service?
    a) solicit input from clients
    b) find out what the competition offers
    c) join a professional network
    d) ignore all criticism

    D

31. A wrapping treatment can be used for:
    a) treating cellulite   c) light exfoliation
    b) firming the skin   d) all of the above are correct

    D

32. Gommage is a French word that means:
    a) to cure   c) to erase
    b) to moisturize   d) to brush

    C

33. How is the grommage product removed from the body?
    a) wiped off with a towel
    b) washed off with water
    c) brushed off with a loofah mitt
    d) rolled off through a friction process

    D

34. Gommage exfoliation is particularly well-suited for what type of environment?
    a) a dry room   c) a dark room
    b) a wet room   d) a bright room

    A

35. What is another term for body wrap?
    a) body polish   c) gommage
    b) body mask   d) exfoliation

    B

36. Some consumers mistakenly believe that all body wraps cause:
    a) weight loss   c) ingrown hairs
    b) premature aging   d) acne

    A

37. Which of the following is a typical product used for a detox treatment?
    a) petroleum jelly   c) milk
    b) shea butter   d) seaweed

    D

38. What are the general categories of algae?
    a) green, blue-green, and brown
    b) green, blue-green, brown, and red
    c) green, blue-green, yellow, and red
    d) green and blue-green

    B

39. Properties of algae include:
    a) skin-restructuring proteins
    b) assistance in cell renewal
    c) metabolic stimulation
    d) all of the above are correct

    D

40. Manufacturers of mud and clay used in mud treatments are required by law to test for:
    a) contaminants
    b) bacteria
    c) toxicity levels
    d) all of the above are correct

    D

41. What is another term for moor mud?
    a) Moroccan mud
    b) peat mud
    c) body mud
    d) organic mud

    B

42. The practice of aromatherapy dates back to:
    a) the Romans
    b) the ancient Egyptians
    c) the ancient Maya
    d) the Vikings

    B

43. A pure blend of essential oils is:
    a) less powerful than a single essential oil
    b) more powerful than a single essential oil
    c) impossible to achieve
    d) a fun thing to experiment with

    B

44. What are essential oils?
    a) a blend of flower aromas and alcohol in a distilled water base
    b) plant extracts
    c) any relaxing oil essential to client care at your spa
    d) none of the above is correct

    B

45. Essential oils contain:
    a) small, tea leaf-size pieces of the plant they came from
    b) a high fat ratio
    c) antiseptics, antibiotics, vitamins, and/or hormones
    d) the same ingredients as many cooking oils

    C

46. The three categories of essential oils used in day spas are:
    a) calming, stimulating, and detoxifying
    b) calming, cheering, and relaxing
    c) energizing, aromatic, and medicinal
    d) extra-oily, medium, and dry

    A

47. An activator is:
    a) a chemical agent used to start the action of chemical products on hair
    b) an additive used to quicken the action or progress of a chemical
    c) another word for booster, accelerator, or catalyst
    d) all of the above are correct

    D

48. Performance agents are:
    a) ingredients that dye skin
    b) ingredients used to obtain an end result
    c) spa personnel who supervise daily performance
    d) not used in spa work

    B

49. Serums are:
    a) not the same as concentrates
    b) only effective if used in large amounts
    c) cost-prohibitive in body treatments
    d) all of the above are correct

    C

50. Finishing lotions, creams, or oils:
    a) must always be applied immediately following treatments
    b) can have fishy or ocean-like smells due to their seaweed content
    c) should be immediately showered off by the client
    d) none of the above is correct

    D

51. Body services:
    a) are in demand to relieve stress
    b) have been around since the early Egyptians
    c) cleanse, exfoliate, treat the skin, and offer stimulation
    d) all of the above are correct

    D

52. What is a salt glow?
    a) the shiny effect of salt on the skin
    b) salt exfoliation
    c) aromatherapy using salt
    d) none of the above is correct

    B

Chapter 34

BODY TREATMENTS

1. The number one priority in performing body treatments is:
   a) completing the treatment
   b) collecting the payment for the service
   c) the safety and well-being of the client
   d) marketing

   C

2. Which of the following products is used for skin conditioning?
   a) gommage
   b) hyaluronic acid serum
   c) shea butter
   d) all of the above are correct

   D

3. How long does a single skin treatment usually take?
   a) 10 minutes
   b) 15 minutes
   c) 25 minutes
   d) one hour

   C

4. How do all body treatments begin?
   a) discussion of costs
   b) massage
   c) initial client consultation
   d) the client is offered a cup of green tea

   C

5. Body treatments involve:
   a) the entire body
   b) only the upper torso
   c) only the extremities
   d) only the lower half of the body

   A

6. The three main goals of a body treatment are:
   a) exfoliation, skin conditioning, and metabolic stimulation
   b) exfoliation, skin conditioning, and relaxation
   c) skin conditioning, metabolic stimulation, and relaxation
   d) skin conditioning, metabolic stimulation, and weight loss

   A

7. Some body treatments are NOT appropriate for:
   a) clients with claustrophobia
   b) pregnant women
   c) clients with open cuts or wounds
   d) all of the above are correct

   D

8. How long should the client rest after the body is wrapped for skin conditioning?
   a) 5 minutes
   b) 10 minutes
   c) 15 minutes
   d) 25 minutes

   B

9. Which of the following types of seaweed is NOT used for a remineralizing seaweed wrap?
   a) green
   b) blue-green
   c) red
   d) brown

   D

10. How do you remove a remineralizing seaweed wrap?
    a) shower or hot towels
    b) loofah brush
    c) rubbing with hands
    d) petroleum jelly

    A

11. What does a detoxifying seaweed wrap use to stimulate and detoxify the body?
    a) water
    b) fish oil
    c) heat
    d) none of the above are correct

    C

12. Which product is more likely to stain, mud or seaweed?
    a) seaweed
    b) mud
    c) both are equally likely to stain
    d) neither will stain

    B

13. What should the client do periodically throughout a remineralizing mud wrap?
    a) sip water
    b) get up and walk around
    c) sleep
    d) stretch the arms

    A

14. Where is an herbal wrap normally performed?
    a) a small room
    b) a large room
    c) a very bright room
    d) a steam room

    B

15. What are spot treatments?
    a) full-body treatments
    b) aromatherapy
    c) localized treatments
    d) none of the above are correct

    C

16. What device is required to perform an herbal wrap?
    a) humidifier
    c) space heater
    b) hydroculator
    d) heating pad

    B

17. For an herbal wrap, the client remains wrapped for up to:
    a) 10 minutes
    c) 20 minutes
    b) 15 minutes
    d) 30 minutes

    C

18. A hand and arm paraffin mask is an example of:
    a) an herbal wrap
    c) a massage
    b) a spot treatment
    d) aromatherapy

    B

19. A back facial is performed by:
    a) a massage therapist
    c) an esthetician
    b) a physical therapist
    d) a dermatologist

    C

20. A spot back treatment is performed by:
    a) a massage therapist
    c) a physical therapist
    b) an esthetician
    d) a dermatologist

    A

21. Which of the following statements about cellulite is NOT true?
    a) Cellulite is a condition that is genetically inherited.
    b) Hormonal changes such as pregnancy or menopause can trigger cellulite.
    c) Cellulite occurs only in obese individuals.
    d) Cellulite never completely goes away.

    C

22. Which of the following is used to treat cellulite?
    a) liposuction
    c) spa treatments
    b) endermology
    d) all of the above are correct

    D

23. In-spa cellulite treatments are scheduled for:
    a) once a week for four to six weeks
    b) twice a week for four to six weeks
    c) twice a week for six to eight weeks
    d) twice a week for eight to ten weeks

    B

24. What is the final step in a cellulite treatment?
    a) Firming cream is applied and massaged into the treated area(s).
    b) A salt scrub is performed to stimulate circulation.
    c) An anticellulite product is applied and massaged into the areas with cellulite.
    d) A detoxifying mask is performed.

    A

25. Which of the following combination treatments is used for cellulite?
    a) cellulite spot treatment with exfoliation
    b) cellulite spot treatment with aromatherapy
    c) cellulite spot treatment with spot back treatment
    d) cellulite spot treatment with full body detox

    D

26. Which of the following treatment choices are used for hand and foot spa treatments?
    a) salt glow   c) aromatherapy massage
    b) seaweed wrap   d) all of the above are correct

    D

27. Most hand and foot treatments should last no longer than:
    a) 15 minutes   c) 45 minutes
    b) 25 minutes   d) one hour

    B

28. Which of the following is a contraindication for a foot treatment?
    a) extra dry skin   c) age spots
    b) fungus   d) whitening

    B

29. Which of the following statements about paraffin treatments is NOT true?
    a) Estheticians apply more layers of paraffin in the summer than in the winter.
    b) Paraffin can be applied over a mud or seaweed mask.
    c) Hospitals have used paraffin for treating arthritis pain.
    d) Paraffin warms the skin.

    A

30. Paraffin should be removed from the body with:
    a) a loofah brush   c) petroleum jelly
    b) an electric mitt   d) hot towels

    D

31. Which of the following statements about paraffin treatments is NOT true?
    a) Paraffin moisturizes the skin.
    b) Paraffin softens the skin.
    c) Paraffin thickens the skin.
    d) Paraffin helps infuse ingredients.

    C

32. How long should a combination hydrotherapy tub and massage take?
    a) 30 minutes
    b) 40 minutes
    c) 50 minutes
    d) one hour

    C

33. How long should a combination hydrotherapy tub, wrap, and massage take?
    a) 50 minutes
    b) one hour
    c) 75 minutes
    d) 90 minutes

    C

34. How long should a combination cellulite treatment and full body detox take?
    a) 30 minutes
    b) 50 minutes
    c) one hour
    d) 75 minutes

    B

35. The benefits of massage include:
    a) relaxes the client
    b) relieves tension and soreness in the client's muscles
    c) energizes the client
    d) all of the above are correct

    D

36. What is effleurage?
    a) a Swedish massage movement in which aggressive kneading activates muscle fiber
    b) a Swedish massage movement in which gentle but firm stroking relaxes the body
    c) a form of hydrotherapy that originated in France
    d) a form of aromatherapy that originated in France

    B

37. What is the specific purpose of percussion in body massage?
    a) to activate nerve endings
    b) to loosen congestion in the lungs
    c) to wake up the client
    d) to relax the client

    A

38. When facing the client, you typically begin a massage:
    a) to your right
    b) to your left
    c) from the top
    d) There is no typical routine for massage.

    B

39. Massage or body treatment is NOT recommended for:
    a) clients with systemic disease   c) diabetics
    b) chemotherapy patients   d) all of the above are correct

    D

40. When pressure is applied to motor points, the body releases:
    a) hormones   c) endorphins
    b) perspiration   d) all of the above are correct

    C

41. The types of massage include:
    a) shiatsu   c) ayurvedic massage
    b) reflexology   d) all of the above are correct

    D

42. What are chakras?
    a) ayurvedic massage energy zones
    b) shiatsu and reflexology energy zones
    c) shiatsu and reflexology energy pathways
    d) ayurvedic massage and treatment energy pathways

    A

43. Shiatsu is a Japanese word that means:
    a) palm pressure therapy
    b) hand pressure therapy
    c) finger pressure therapy
    d) Shiatsu is actually the Chinese word for massage.

    C

44. The key to a successful shiatsu treatment is:
    a) applying great pressure on a stressed motor point to relieve stress
    b) applying pressure smoothly and evenly and relieving stress in a painless way
    c) applying very light pressure on stressed motor points to relieve stress
    d) applying pressure only from the fingertips

    B

45. Pressing the client's temples in a facial massage is an example of
    a) reflexology   c) ayurvedic massage
    b) shiatsu   d) Swedish massage

    B

46. The focus of reflexology is solely on:
    a) the face
    b) the back
    c) the feet and hands
    d) the legs

    C

47. Who coined the term reflexology?
    a) Joe Shelby Riley
    b) Eunice Inghram
    c) Albert Einstein
    d) The derivation of the term is unknown.

    B

48. The categories of body products sold by spas or salons include:
    a) professionally designed soap
    b) shower gel or foam bath
    c) body lotions and creams
    d) all of the above are correct

    D

49. Besides reducing cellulite, what is a major result of cellulite treatments?
    a) reduces water retention
    b) removes ingrown hairs
    c) hydrates the body
    d) increases electrolytes

    A

Chapter 35

CAREER OPPORTUNITIES IN MEDICAL ESTHETICS

1. A new area of involvement for estheticians in recent years is:
   a) the sports arena
   b) the medical arena
   c) bioethics
   d) the diet industry

   B

2. Which of the following statements about medical esthetics is true?
   a) Medical esthetics means to integrate surgical procedures and esthetic treatments.
   b) Medical esthetics supports demands for long-term age-management programs.
   c) Including medical esthetics in your business is a good way to increase profits.
   d) all of the above are correct

   D

3. What explains the emergence of medical esthetics?
   a) patient interest
   b) the improvement in skin care treatment
   c) the issue of liability
   d) new legislation

   B

4. What should medical estheticians learn in their first few months at school?
   a) cosmetic chemistry
   b) camouflage techniques
   c) basic business skills
   d) all of the above are correct

   D

5. In which of the following medical settings can you encounter an esthetician?
   a) medical spa
   b) laser center
   c) hospital
   d) all of the above are correct

   D

6. What determines the responsibilities of your position?
   a) your training
   b) the individual setting
   c) state laws
   d) all of the above are correct

   B

7. What is an ancillary profit center?
   a) a medical spa that treats only hands and feet
   b) a medical office that is making a profit
   c) a separate profit-generating department within the medical office
   d) a cosmetic surgeon's office

   C

8. In which setting are you likely to assist in clinical studies?
   a) cosmetic surgeon's office
   b) dermatology office
   c) outpatient clinic
   d) medi-spa

   B

9. Which of the following procedures can be perfomed by an esthetician working in a dermatology office?
   a) routine facial
   b) extraction
   c) microdermabrasion
   d) all of the above are correct

   D

10. In which setting is it particularly important for the esthetician to possess advanced knowledge of major malpractice and liability insurance?
    a) independent clinic
    b) hospital
    c) laser center
    d) dermatology office

    A

11. Which of the following is NOT a patient educator's responsibility?
    a) ensure that the patient follows home care instructions
    b) ensure that the patient comes to appointments
    c) establish product protocols
    d) all of the above are a patient educator's responsibility

    D

12. Which of the following procedures is NOT performed at a laser center?
    a) spider vein removal
    b) collagen injection
    c) nonablative wrinkle treatment
    d) laser hair reduction

    B

13. Which of the following statements about collagen injections is NOT true?
    a) A collagen injection is a filler, usually bovine derivative.
    b) A collagen injection makes lips larger.
    c) A collagen injection removes age spots.
    d) A collagen injection fills in wrinkles.

    C

14. In what setting would an esthetician most likely manage a retail area?
    a) dermatology office
    b) cosmetic surgeon's office
    c) hospital
    d) Retail areas do not exist in medical settings.

    C

15. A medical team can include:
    a) nurse practitioners
    b) massage therapists
    c) licensed estheticians
    d) all of the above are correct

    D

16. What should you NOT do before beginning a job search?
    a) Access career counseling services at your school.
    b) Access job placement services at your school.
    c) Define the kind of setting you would like to work in.
    d) Impress prospective employers by spontaneously visiting them at their office before submitting a resume.

    D

17. What is the first step in forming a good resume?
    a) take a class on how to write a resume
    b) discuss your goals with a career counselor
    c) get organized
    d) prepare a list of solid references

    C

18. What is the most important tool you need to create a good resume?
    a) fine bond paper
    b) a good how-to manual
    c) a computer
    d) a good printer

    C

19. Good resumes are:
    a) brief
    b) tailored to meet particular job requirements
    c) prepared in several formats
    d) all of the above are correct

    D

20. Which of the following is NOT usually provided in resumes?
    a) your career objective
    b) your birth date
    c) a history of your experience
    d) awards or achievements

    B

21. The tasks and duties of an esthetician working in a cosmetic surgeon's office do NOT usually include:
    a) research
    b) laser hair reduction
    c) pre- and postop care
    d) managing a retail center

    A

22. The tasks and duties of an esthetician working in an outpatient clinic do NOT usually include:
    a) patient education
    b) camouflage therapy
    c) endermology
    d) laser hair reduction

    C

23. The tasks and duties of an esthetician working in a hospital do NOT usually include:
    a) patient education
    b) research
    c) laser hair reduction
    d) training

    D

24. The tasks and duties of an esthetician working in an independent clinic do NOT usually include:
    a) patient education
    b) clinic administration
    c) training
    d) managing a retail center

    A

25. The tasks and duties of an esthetician working in a laser center do NOT usually include:
    a) administering laser therapy
    b) patient education
    c) administering light therapy
    d) research

    D

26. The tasks and duties of an esthetician working in a cosmetic dentist's office do NOT usually include:
    a) camouflage therapy
    b) product sales
    c) managing a retail center
    d) routine skin care

    A

27. The tasks and duties of an esthetician working in a medical spa do NOT usually include:
    a) laser therapy
    b) endermology
    c) training
    d) routine skin care

    C

28. What is the compensation for a medical esthetician in a cosmetic physician's office?
    a) $10 to $15 hourly plus 15% to 20% commission on product sales and treatments
    b) $15 to $20 hourly plus 20% to 30% commission on product sales and treatments
    c) $12 to $30 hourly plus 15% to 30% commission on product sales and treatments
    d) $20 to $35 hourly plus 15% to 30% commission on product sales and treatments

    C

29. What is the compensation for a medical esthetician in a derma-
    tology office?
    a) $12 to $25 hourly plus 15% to 20% commission on product sales and
       treatments
    b) $12 to $25 hourly
    c) $15 to $25 hourly
    d) $20 to $35 hourly plus 15% commission on product sales
       and treatments

     C

30. What is the compensation for a medical esthetician in an outpa-
    tient clinic?
    a) $20 to $30 hourly
    b) $15 to $25 hourly plus 15% to 50% commission on product
       sales and treatments
    c) $12 to $25 hourly plus 15% to 30% commission on product
       sales and treatments
    d) $20 to $35 hourly plus 15% to 25% commission on product
       sales and treatments

     B

31. What is the compensation for a medical esthetician in a hospital?
    a) $15 to $25 hourly
    b) $12 to $20 hourly
    c) $20 to $30 hourly
    d) $12 to $15 hourly plus 15% to 30% commission on product
       sales and treatments

     A

32. What is the compensation for a medical esthetician in an inde-
    pendent clinic?
    a) $20 to $30 hourly
    b) $15 to $50 hourly
    c) $15 to $50 hourly plus commission on product sales and treatments
    d) $15 to $25 hourly plus 15% to 50% commission on product
       sales and treatments

     C

33. What is the compensation for a medical esthetician in a laser
    center?
    a) $20 to $30 hourly
    b) $12 to $20 hourly
    c) $15 to $20 hourly
    d) $15 to $25 hourly plus 15% to 25% commission on product
       sales and treatments

    B

34. What is the compensation for a medical esthetician in a cosmetic dentist's office?
    a) $12 to $15 hourly plus 15% to 25% commission on product sales
    b) $15 to $25 hourly plus 15% to 30% commission on product sales
    c) $20 to $30 hourly
    d) $20 to $35 hourly plus 15% to 25% commission on product sales

35. What is the compensation for a medical esthetician in a medical spa?
    a) $15 to $30 hourly
    b) $15 to $30 hourly plus commission on product sales
    c) $20 to $30 hourly
    d) $20 to $30 hourly plus 15% to 25% commission on product sales and treatments

Chapter 36

PLASTIC AND RECONSTRUCTIVE SURGERY

1. The "plastic" in plastic surgery means:
   a) hard, durable, and expensive
   b) fit for molding, malleable, moldable
   c) artificial
   d) temporary

   B

2. Which of the following is NOT a specialty in cosmetic surgery?
   a) plastic surgery
   b) dermatology
   c) reconstructive plastic surgery
   d) arthroscopic surgery

   D

3. A facial plastic surgeon is board certified in:
   a) opthamology
   b) cosmetic dentistry
   c) otolaryngology
   d) Board certification is not required.

   C

4. Dermatologists specialize in disorders and diseases of:
   a) skin
   b) hair
   c) nails
   d) all of the above are correct

   D

5. Networking does NOT involve:
   a) honing your hard-sell skills
   b) setting goals thoughtfully
   c) taking part in community, business, and charity events
   d) keeping a notebook and/or calendar

   A

6. Common facial plastic surgery procedures do NOT include:
   a) needle biopsy
   b) otoplasty
   c) laser resurfacing
   d) phenol peel

   A

7. A face-lift does NOT:
    a) remove excess fat at the jaw line
    b) tighten loose, atrophic muscles
    c) remove sagging, draping skin
    d) improve breathing by clearing and widening nasal and
       tracheal passages

    D

8. Another word for face-lift is:
    a) rhytidectomy   c) rhinocortisone
    b) rhinoplasty   d) rhizotomy

    A

9. Where are face-lift incisions located?
    a) behind and around the ear and hairline
    b) beneath the chin
    c) inside the mouth
    d) location varies according to each patient

    A

10. The forehead lift is NOT:
    a) called the brow lift
    b) known as otoplasty
    c) historically part of the face-lift but now performed separately
    d) performed to lift a sagging forehead

    B

11. The forehead lift does NOT:
    a) tighten muscles   c) remove excess skin
    b) lift excess skin   d) reduce hair loss

    D

12. Blepharoplasty is:
    a) the removal of facial blemishes through any chemical peel
    b) an eyelift
    c) the injection of collagen into the lips
    d) There is no such procedure.

    B

13. An eyelift does NOT:
    a) remove fat from eyelids
    b) involve the upper lid, lower lid, or both
    c) improve eyesight
    d) remove skin from eyelid

    C

14. The forehead lift is performed:
    a) at any spa, usually during a wrap or massage
    b) in the client's home
    c) with the client under general anesthesia
    d) over several sessions lasting up to six months

    C

15. Rhinoplasty is NOT:
    a) another word for nose surgery
    b) performed to change the shape of the nose
    c) a firming agent used in nose surgeries
    d) sometimes needed to improve nasal function

 C

16. Otoplasty is NOT:
    a) a procedure performed to flatten ears
    b) another name for all plastic surgeries
    c) a procedure requiring general anesthesia
    d) often performed on children

 B

17. Transconjunctival blepharoplasty:
    a) is a procedure performed inside the lower eyelid
    b) involves transferring tissue from one part of the eyelid to another
    c) is performed in conjunction with blemish removal
    d) is no longer performed in this country

 A

18. Laser is an acronym for:
    a) long-acting surgical-effect radiation
    b) holograms
    c) light amplification by the stimulated emission of radiation
    d) laser is not an acronym

C

19. Laser resurfacing does NOT:
    a) smooth wrinkles   c) vaporize skin
    b) cure acne   d) soften or lessen old acne scars

 B

20. Collagen remodeling is:
    a) the stimulation of the growth of new collagen in the dermis
    b) the relocating of collagen from one area of the face to another
    c) never used with lasers
    d) a procedure performed on collagen before it is injected

A

21. Side effects of laser surgery do NOT include:
    a) hypopigmentation
    b) recombination of DNA at the molecular level
    c) hyperpigmentation
    d) changes in skin color

 B

 22. Trichloroacetic Acid Peels (TCA) are NOT recommended for:
    a) sun damage   c) semi-annual follow-ups to face-lifts
    b) wrinkles   d) precancerous lesions

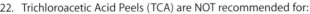 C

23. Patients with what skin types are good candidates for TCA?
    a) darker skin pigments
    c) Fitzpatrick types III and IV
    b) all Fitzpatrick types
    d) no Fitzpatrick types

    C

24. Phenol peels are NOT:
    a) used less often than in previous decades
    b) potentially toxic
    c) available for sale in spas for home use
    d) less expensive than laser treatments

    C

25. A mammaplasty is NOT:
    a) breast augmentation
    b) most easily performed with lasers
    c) a plastic surgery body procedure
    d) performed on an anesthetized patient

    B

26. The most common area of incision in mammaplasty is:
    a) the endoscopic cavity
    b) beneath the chest muscle
    c) the top of the breast
    d) this procedure requires no incisions

    B

27. Gynecomastia is:
    a) the excessive development of the male mammary glands
    b) the excessive development of the female mammary glands
    c) infection resulting from saline implants
    d) breast augmentation

    A

28. The transumbilical method is a breast augmentation procedure in which the incision is made:
    a) under the breast fold
    c) through the navel
    b) in the ambulacrum
    d) through the armpit

    C

29. Which of the following procedures is NOT performed under general anesthesia?
    a) the transumbilical method
    c) abdominoplasty
    b) Botox treatment
    d) phenol peel

    B

30. Common problems associated with enlarged breasts include:
    a) difficulty breathing
    c) back problems
    b) restricted activity
    d) all of the above are correct

    D

31. Which of the following is NOT an area of the body treated with liposuction?
    a) stomach
    b) jaw line
    c) feet
    d) arms

    _C_

32. Types of anesthesia used for liposuction include:
    a) local
    b) IV
    c) general
    d) all of the above are correct

    _D_

33. Abdominoplasty is:
    a) liposuction on the stomach
    b) fat deposits and loose skin in the abdomen are tucked and tightened
    c) laser surgery performed on skin in the abdomen
    d) collagen injections in the abdomen

    _B_

34. How is the skin affected by abdominoplasty?
    a) it is drawn up
    b) it is drawn down
    c) blemishes are removed
    d) skin is loosened

    _B_

35. Methods of liposuction include:
    a) liposuction with general anesthesia
    b) tumescent liposuction
    c) ultrasonic lipoplasty
    d) all of the above are correct

    _D_

36. The areola is:
    a) the armpit
    b) the breast fold
    c) the nipple
    d) the incision site in breast augmentation surgery

    _C_

37. The axilla is:
    a) the incision scar
    b) the armpit
    c) the liposuction tool
    d) the breast fold

    _B_

38. What is an endoscope?
    a) a long tube with a light on the end
    b) a short tube with a light on the end
    c) a laser
    d) a scalpel

    _A_

39. Maxillofacial surgeons specialize in treating:
    a) the eyes
    b) the nose
    c) the mouth and jaw
    d) the ears

    C

40. Which of the following is NOT treated with Botox?
    a) excessive perspiration
    b) migraines
    c) excessive muscle stretching
    d) crow's feet

    C

41. How does a Botox treatment affect the muscle?
    a) improves the muscle's ability to function
    b) mitigates the muscle's ability to function
    c) repairs tears in the muscle
    d) strengthens the muscle

    B

42. What is Botox created from?
    a) animal tissue
    b) plants
    c) a bacterium
    d) none of the above are correct

    C

43. Which of the following is NOT performed under a <u>local</u> anesthetic:
    a) spider vein removal
    b) Botox treatment
    c) forehead lift
    d) nonablative wrinkle treatment

    C

44. Ligation is:
    a) removing veins
    b) tying off veins
    c) unblocking veins
    d) taking legal action

    B

45. Sclerotherapy is a procedure that helps remove:
    a) medium-size veins
    b) very large veins
    c) small veins
    d) spider veins

    A

46. Which of the following conditions is NOT treated with radio frequency?
    a) spider veins
    b) bulging veins
    c) warts
    d) skin cancers

    B

47. A phlebectomy does what to the bulging vein protruding above the skin's surface?
    a) makes a large incision
    b) makes very small incisions
    c) eradicates it with a laser
    d) ties off the vein

    B

48. In what decade were phlebectomies first performed in the United States?
    a) 1960s
    b) 1970s
    c) 1980s
    d) 1990s

    D

49. What does the patient normally have to wear following sclerotherapy?
    a) bandages
    b) compression hose
    c) cotton pants
    d) special shoes

    B

50. Which of the following conditions is NOT treated with a collagen filler?
    a) chickenpox scars
    b) migraine headaches
    c) crow's feet
    d) deep furrows in forehead

    B

51. Spider veins can appear on:
    a) the face
    b) legs
    c) ankles
    d) all of the above are correct

    D

52. Spider veins are also called:
    a) varicose veins
    b) sclerotic veins
    c) telangiectasia
    d) none of the above are correct

    C

53. In place of which procedure is ligation sometimes performed?
    a) ambulatory phlebectomy
    b) sclerotherapy
    c) radio frequency
    d) laser hair reduction

    A

54. How long does it take to perform laser hair reduction?
    a) one hour
    b) a few minutes
    c) two hours
    d) 30 minutes

    B

55. How much training is required to perform laser hair reduction?
    a) minimal
    b) advanced
    c) moderate
    d) varies from state to state

    B

56. What type of anesthesia is used for a nonablative wrinkle treatment?
    a) IV
    b) general
    c) local
    d) no anesthesia

    D

57. How many types of plastic surgery are there?
    a) one
    b) two
    c) three
    d) four

    B

58. Which of the following is considered a "traditional" plastic surgery procedure?
    a) tummy tuck
    b) laser resurfacing
    c) chemical peel
    d) nonablative wrinkle treatment

    A

59. Which of the following procedures are relatively new?
    a) laser resurfacing
    b) chemical peels
    c) nonablative wrinkle treatments
    d) all of the above are correct

    D

60. What is another name for cosmetic surgery?
    a) aesthetic surgery
    b) facial surgery
    c) rhytidectomy
    d) elective surgery

    A

61. A dermatologist is board certified in:
    a) endocrinolgy
    b) opthamology
    c) dermatology
    d) Board certification is not required.

    C

62. Which of the following is a professional organization of dermatologists in the U.S.?
    a) American Society of Dermatologists
    b) American Academy of Dermatology
    c) American Association of Dermatology
    d) American Dermatology Guild

    B

63. TMJ is a disorder of the jaw caused by:
    a) stress
    b) injury
    c) disease
    d) all of the above are correct

    D

64. What condition do you have if you undergo Mohs' micrographic surgery?
    a) skin cancer
    b) TMJ
    c) breathing problems
    d) spider veins

    A

65. Which of the following is a procedure often performed on children?
    a) rhinoplasty
    b) otoplasty
    c) blepharoplasty
    d) laser resurfacing

    B

66. Which of the following is a type of laser?
    a) collagen laser
    b) erbium laser
    c) endoscopic laser
    d) axilla laser

67. Until the 1990s, phenol was widely used for:
    a) cleaning the skin
    b) smoothing and retexturizing the skin
    c) laser resurfacing
    d) remove old acne scars

Chapter 37

PATIENT PROFILES

1. The five types of patients most often encountered include:
   a) survivors of domestic violence
   b) pre- and postoperative patients
   c) elderly
   d) all of the above are correct _____

2. How do preoperative patients tend to feel about their upcoming procedure?
   a) calm   c) angry
   b) nervous   d) delighted _____

3. Approximately how long after surgery should the esthetician wait to perform therapies on the postoperative patient?
   a) 2 days   b) 2 weeks
   a) 1 week   c) 2 months _____

4. In dealing with survivors of domestic abuse, with whom should the esthetician maintain an open dialog at all times?
   a) the physican   c) a Social Services counselor
   b) her supervisor   d) the pyschologist _____

5. Guidelines for dealing with survivors of abuse do NOT include:
   a) asking patients how they sustained their injuries
   b) explaining to patients exactly what you can do for them
   c) working in partnership with the patient's physician
   d) all of the above are correct _____

6. Guidelines for elderly patients include:
   a) letting them know you don't think they are being vain
   b) using clear language when explaining a treatment
   c) sharing samples appropriate for their skin type even if they choose not to buy
   d) all of the above are correct   _____

7. When working with the physically challenged do NOT:
   a) make daily rituals as easy as possible
   b) say "It's easy, just do..."
   c) change the room around to make access easy for the patient
   d) remember a degenerative disability may have worsened _____

8. Which of the below are possible indications of mental illness?
   a) many open wounds, yet no real interest in a skin care program
   b) inability to cope, crying, or extreme behavior
   c) deep scars
   d) all of the above are correct   _____

9. What should you do if you observe signs of mental illness in a client?
   a) perform the treatment the client wants
   b) call a hospital
   c) do not perform any treatment and refer the client to a physician
   d) none of the above is correct   _____

10. A complete surgical plan for the pre- and postoperative patient does NOT include:
    a) consultation   c) actual surgery
    b) meeting with the surgeon d) procedure education   _____

11. Which is a key factor in building a relationship with a patient?
    a) consultation with their physician
    b) supervisor consultation
    c) patient consultation
    d) none of the above are correct   _____

12. Home care compliance is extremely important because:
    a) it does not support surgical results
    b) it does not expedite the healing process
    c) both a and b are correct
    d) neither a nor b is correct   _____

13. Who is an ideal candidate for an elective surgery?
    a) only elderly patients
    b) anyone who can afford it
    c) someone who has realistic expectations
    d) someone who's parent has made the decision for them _____

14. Which is an important issue in patient selection?
    a) personality match   c) conditioning
    b) compliance   d) intimidation _____

15. Teaching or instructing the patient with the necessary protocols to ensure a positive surgical outcome is called:
    a) patient education   c) SOAP notes
    b) home care compliance   d) charting _____

16. Coding preoperative protocols in one color and postoperative protocols in another is an example of what concept in teaching?
    a) Socratic method   c) compliance
    b) show and tell   d) SOAP notes _____

17. Arranging skin care products sequentially on a tray and in different sized containers is a method for helping:
    a) elderly patients   c) mentally unstable patients
    b) hearing-impaired patients d) visually-impaired patients _____

18. Taking care of yourself might include:
    a) daily breaks away from the office
    b) yoga class
    c) finding a mentor or support person
    d) all of the above are correct _____

19. A client's medical chart is:
    a) often incomplete   c) a public document
    b) confidential   d) none of the above
                                     are correct _____

20. Release of any information is allowed only with the written consent of the:
    a) esthetician   c) patient
    b) physician   d) spa owner _____

21. SOAP stands for:
    a) Standard Operations And Procedures
    b) Standard Operations And Protocols
    c) Subjective, Objective, Assessment, Protocol
    d) Subjective, Objective, Assessment, Plan   _____

22. In chart writing, describing the problem from the patient's per-
    spective is called:
    a) subjective data   c) assessment
    b) objective data   d) planning   _____

23. A conclusion reached on the basis of data is called:
    a) subjective data   c) assessment
    b) objective data   d) planning   _____

24. Describing what you see without making a judgement is called:
    a) subjective data   c) assessment
    b) objective data   d) planning   _____

25. Since protocols are not standardized throughout the skin care
    industry, when documenting procedures, estheticians should
    use:
    a) careful notes   c) SOAP notes
    b) the SOP manual   d) consent forms   _____

26. Which is NOT a standard protocol for a glycolic peel?
    a) signing a consent form
    b) applying eye covers
    c) applying sunscreen
    d) referring the client to a physician   _____

27. How often should you share information with the client's physi-
    cian during the pre- and postsurgery time frame?
    a) routinely   c) twice
    b) once   d) only in emergencies   _____

28. If you are uncomfortable dealing with certain issues while treat-
    ing a patient, it is perfectly appropriate to withhold treatment
    and refer the patient back to the physician or to another profes-
    sional for assistance. This statement is:
    a) sometimes true   c) never true
    b) always true   d) rarely true   _____

29. A legal document stating that the patient agrees to the treatment and understands and accepts all risks involved is called:
    a) a consultation form
    b) a home care guide
    c) an informed consent form
    d) a protocol
    _____

30. The most important business tool estheticians have is:
    a) voicemail
    b) the telephone
    c) a mailing list
    d) technology
    _____

31. Telephone etiquette includes which rule(s)?
    a) don't make them wait
    b) return calls promptly
    c) a little courtesy goes a long way
    d) all of the above are correct
    _____

32. Your business phone should be answered within how many rings?
    a) two
    b) three
    c) four
    d) five
    _____

33. What should you do before placing a client on hold?
    a) ask their permission to do so
    b) take their name and number
    c) say hello quickly and tell them to hold
    d) ask them to call back if you get disconnected
    _____

34. What should your voicemail recording say in order to be user-friendly?
    a) the name of your company and the hours of business
    b) when you plan to return calls
    c) both a and b are correct
    d) neither a nor b is correct
    _____

35. Calls should be returned within what time frame, realistically?
    a) two hours
    b) twenty-four hours
    c) forty-eight hours
    d) one week
    _____

36. A method used to assist patients who are visually impaired by using a CD or cassette tape recorder to verbalize information is called:
    a) show don't tell
    b) auditory
    c) oratory
    d) protocol
    _____

37. Drugs that penetrate beyond the epidermis and are prescription only are called:
    a) topical
    b) active agents
    c) inactive agents
    d) irritants   _____

38. Consent forms for peels and microdermabrasion have which in common?
    a) they state there is no guarantee
    b) they ask for the patient's signature
    c) they ask for the esthetician's signature
    d) all of the above are correct   _____

39. Is it ever appropriate to experiment with a new treatment or product on a client?
    a) yes, always
    b) no, never
    c) yes, if the client agrees
    d) yes, if authorized to do so by the physician   _____

40. The purpose of the intake questionnaire is to:
    a) learn as much as possible about the health of the skin
    b) aid in providing services safely and effectively
    c) uncover the client's needs and wants
    d) all of the above are correct   _____

Chapter 38

PRE- AND POSTOPERATIVE CARE

1. In the preoperative phase, conditioning the skin to heal does
   NOT include:
   a) increasing the skin's metabolism
   b) reducing cellular debris
   c) decreasing inflammation
   d) all of the above are correct   _____

2. Surgery results are highly dependent on:
   a) the patient's willingness to follow all protocols
   b) the patient's willingness to abandon all protocols
   c) the patient's ability to abandon all prior routines
   d) none of the above are correct   _____

3. Why should clients have skin treatments prior to surgery?
   a) to make the surgeon's job easier
   b) to optimize the patient's tolerance for the postoperative phase
   c) to see if surgery is really necessary
   d) they shouldn't; only postoperative treatments are necessary   _____

4. A blepharoplasty is the medical term for:
   a) a facelift   c) a forehead lift
   b) an eyelift   d) a tummy tuck   _____

5. Ideally, how many weeks before surgery do protocols for a
   rhytidectomy begin?
   a) 8-10   c) 4-5
   b) 5-6   d) 1   _____

6. Which treatment utilizes a series of light rhythmic movements to stimulate lymph fluid flow?
   a) microdermabrasion
   b) alpha hydroxy peels
   c) endermology
   d) manual lymphatic drainage _____

7. When performed preoperatively, MLD's benefits include:
   a) increased hydration
   b) lowered stress levels
   c) detoxification
   d) all of the above are correct _____

8. MLD has its roots in:
   a) India
   b) Japan
   c) Europe
   d) California _____

9. Alpha and beta hydroxy peels are also known as:
   a) lunch-time peels
   b) lunch-pail peels
   c) coffee-break peels
   d) none of the above are correct _____

10. When working with chemical peels, estheticians should work strictly with the:
    a) dermis
    b) epidermis
    c) stratum corneum
    d) epithelius _____

11. The benefits of chemical peels do NOT include:
    a) lifting superficial hyperpigmentation
    b) making skin appear smoother
    c) eliminating dead cellular debris
    d) lifting superficial hypopigmentation _____

12. Exfoliation of the statum corneum through the use of a machine that fires crystals through a hand piece is called:
    a) microdermabrasion
    b) endermology
    c) rhytidectomy
    d) blepharoplasty _____

13. For the patient, benefits of using microdermabrasion include:
    a) it can replace chemicals
    b) it provides an even peel
    c) it takes a limited amount of time
    d) all of the above are correct _____

14. Which procedure does NOT require advanced training?
    a) massage
    b) light peels
    c) microdermabrasion
    d) MLD _____

15. Which is a cellulite treatment given before and after liposuction?
    a) endermology
    b) abdomectomy
    c) rhytidectomy
    d) blepharoplasty
    _____

16. Benefits of a massage do NOT include:
    a) less cellulite
    b) a sense of well-being
    c) improved circulation
    d) reduced stress
    _____

17. Which plays a role in all phases of both pre- and postoperative care, incorporating consultation, education, patient selection, and medical documentation?
    a) microdermabrasion
    b) massage
    c) computer imaging
    d) lunch-time peels
    _____

18. When procedures are combined, the esthetician should:
    a) create a plan for the most difficult procedure
    b) create a plan that uses the easiest protocols for the patient
    c) create a combined treatment plan
    d) defer to a physician for a treatment plan
    _____

19. Nonmedical-grade lighters that can be used as part of the home care plan for preoperative laser resurfacing include:
    a) licorice extract
    b) bearberry
    c) kojic acid
    d) all of the above are correct
    _____

20. Green tea extract, an antioxidant that helps to neutralize free radicals, is used in the home care for which type of care?
    a) preoperative laser resurfacing
    b) postoperative laser resurfacing
    c) preoperative face-lift
    d) postoperative face-lift
    _____

21. How long before surgery should a preoperative laser resurfacing client take anitviral medication to prevent a herpetic breakout?
    a) one day
    b) one week
    c) two weeks
    d) one month
    _____

22. How soon can camouflage therapy begin for the postoperative laser resurfacing client?
    a) 3 months
    b) 15-30 days
    c) 5-10 days
    d) 1-5 days
    _____

23. Metro-gel cream:
    a) reduces redness in rosacea patients
    b) is a topical antibiotic
    c) both a and b are correct
    d) neither a nor b is correct   _____

24. What treatment should be performed every 2-3 days during the week prior to face-lift surgery?
    a) microdermabrasion   c) lymphatic drainage massage
    b) chemical peel   d) swedish massage   _____

25. Which does NOT take place in the first week after face-lift surgery?
    a) Drains are removed.
    b) Bandages are replaced with a facial bra.
    c) Patient comes in for postoperative appointment with physician.
    d) Sutures and staples are removed.   _____

26. How soon after surgery can face-lift patients return to presurgery home care?
    a) 2 weeks   c) 1 month
    b) 3 weeks   d) 6 weeks   _____

27. Which product will help reduce swelling for preoperative eye-lift patients?
    a) hyaluronic acid   c) bioflavonoids
    b) cucumber extract   d) hydroquinone   _____

28. What home care regimen should the esthetician stress for post-operative eye-lift patients during the first week after surgery?
    a) ice   c) Tylenol
    b) eyedrops   d) hydrocortisone   _____

29. MLD should NOT be performed on anyone with:
    a) severe sinusitis   c) basal cell carcinoma
    b) pnemonia   d) all of the above are correct   _____

30. To avoid unnecessary reactions, always do a patch test:
    a) on the elbow   c) on the neck
    b) on the underside of the arm   d) behind the ear   _____

31. What is NOT a recommended way to continue learning after
    your formal training?
    a) alumni organizations   c) vendor presentations
    b) trade associations   d) reading women's magazines _____

32. Contraindications for microdermabrasion include:
    a) varicose veins   c) heart conditions
    b) major circulatory problems d) none of the above
                                     are correct   _____

Chapter *39*

CAMOUFLAGE THERAPY

1. The consistency of camouflage therapy makeup is:
   a) thicker
   b) thinner
   c) similar to any other type of makeup
   d) depends on the brand used _____

2. Why might one need to use camouflage makeup?
   a) to make the nose appear smaller
   b) to make the eyes appear larger
   c) to disguise a congenital disfigurement
   d) to cover up acne _____

3. How soon after a patient receives laser resurfacing will a physician authorize camouflage makeup?
   a) 1-2 days
   b) 5-7 days
   c) 10-14 days
   d) 18-21 days _____

4. What is a rhytidectomy?
   a) an eyelift
   b) bruising of the skin
   c) extreme redness of the skin
   d) a face-lift _____

5. What color of makeup is usually preferred to neutralize redness?
   a) green
   b) blue
   c) tan
   d) yellow _____

6. Which skin condition can receive camouflage therapy?
   a) skin with lesions
   b) skin with bruising
   c) skin with extreme acne
   d) skin with a staph infection _____

7. How should you approach the patient receiving camouflage treatment?
   a) be patient, pleasant, and consistent
   b) be aggressive
   c) be extremely optimistic
   d) be controlling   _____

8. An example of micropigmentation is a:
   a) freckle
   b) tattoo
   c) bruise
   d) mole   _____

9. Micropigmentation has been done since:
   a) 2000 B.C.
   b) 3000 B.C.
   c) 1000 B.C.
   d) 1500 A.D.   _____

10. A typical use for permanent cosmetic makeup is:
    a) hair removal
    b) restore pigment
    c) permanent tan
    d) permanent eyeshadow   _____

Answer
Keys

CHAPTER 1 - A JOURNEY THROUGH TIME: ESTHETICS THEN AND NOW

(Answers to Questions on Pages 1-2)

1-b	4-b	7-d	10-b	13-b
2-c	5-b	8-d	11-d	
3-b	6-a	9-d	12-c	

CHAPTER 2 - ANATOMY AND PHYSIOLOGY OF THE SKIN

(Answers to Questions on Pages 3-11)

1-c	16-d	31-c	46-c	61-a
2-b	17-b	32-d	47-c	62-d
3-c	18-c	33-c	48-d	63-d
4-a	19-c	34-a	49-c	64-c
5-d	20-b	35-c	50-c	65-a
6-c	21-b	36-b	51-a	66-c
7-a	22-a	37-c	52-d	67-b
8-d	23-a	38-c	53-b	68-d
9-c	24-a	39-c	54-c	69-b
10-c	25-a	40-b	55-c	70-c
11-a	26-c	41-c	56-b	71-d
12-b	27-a	42-b	57-b	72-b
13-c	28-b	43-d	58-c	73-a
14-d	29-b	44-a	59-c	74-b
15-a	30-d	45-b	60-d	75-d

CHAPTER 3 - BODY SYSTEMS

(Answers to Questions on Pages 12-15)

1-d	8-b	15-c	22-c	29-a
2-a	9-c	16-d	23-d	30-a
3-c	10-d	17-a	24-b	31-a
4-d	11-d	18-c	25-d	32-d
5-d	12-b	19-b	26-b	
6-a	13-d	20-a	27-d	
7-d	14-b	21-b	28-b	

CHAPTER 4 - BONES, MUSCLES, AND NERVES OF THE FACE AND SKULL

(Answers to Questions on Pages 16-19)

1-c	8-c	15-c	22-b	29-b
2-a	9-a	16-b	23-a	30-b
3-a	10-c	17-a	24-b	31-b
4-c	11-b	18-c	25-b	32-c
5-c	12-c	19-d	26-c	33-d
6-a	13-b	20-a	27-d	34-c
7-c	14-c	21-c	28-b	

CHAPTER 5 - BACTERIOLOGY AND SANITATION

(Answers to Questions on Pages 20-22)

1-c	5-d	9-c	13-d	17-d
2-a	6-c	10-c	14-c	18-b
3-d	7-b	11-d	15-c	19-b
4-a	8-c	12-d	16-a	20-c

CHAPTER 6 - NUTRITION

(Answers to Questions on Pages 23-28)

1-d	10-a	19-b	28-c	37-d
2-a	11-a	20-b	29-b	38-b
3-c	12-d	21-c	30-b	39-c
4-b	13-d	22-d	31-c	40-b
5-d	14-b	23-d	32-d	41-c
6-b	15-b	24-d	33-b	42-d
7-b	16-a	25-d	34-d	43-a
8-c	17-c	26-d	35-d	
9-d	18-c	27-c	36-a	

CHAPTER 7 - ROOM FURNISHINGS

(Answers to Questions on Pages 29-30)

1-a	3-d	5-c	7-a
2-c	4-d	6-d	

CHAPTER 8 - TECHNOLOGICAL TOOLS

(Answers to Questions on Pages 31-38)

1-b	14-d	27-c	40-a	53-c
2-b	15-d	28-d	41-a	54-c
3-a	16-a	29-c	42-c	55-d
4-d	17-b	30-a	43-d	56-a
5-b	18-d	31-d	44-b	57-d
6-d	19-b	32-a	45-b	58-d
7-d	20-b	33-c	46-c	59-a
8-c	21-d	34-a	47-d	60-a
9-d	22-c	35-d	48-d	61-d
10-c	23-c	36-b	49-c	62-b
11-a	24-a	37-a	50-d	63-a
12-d	25-c	38-a	51-d	64-c
13-b	26-c	39-d	52-d	

CHAPTER 9 - BASICS OF ELECTRICITY

(Answers to Questions on Pages 39-44)

1-d	10-d	19-c	28-a	37-d
2-c	11-a	20-c	29-a	38-d
3-b	12-a	21-a	30-b	39-c
4-a	13-b	22-c	31-a	40-d
5-c	14-c	23-c	32-d	41-d
6-d	15-d	24-b	33-b	42-d
7-b	16-d	25-b	34-b	
8-b	17-b	26-c	35-d	
9-b	18-d	27-c	36-d	

CHAPTER 10 - FIRST IMPRESSIONS - SETUP AND SUPPLIES

(Answers to Questions on Pages 45-47)

1-a	5-d	9-d	13-b	17-c
2-d	6-d	10-d	14-c	18-d
3-c	7-c	11-d	15-a	19-b
4-a	8-a	12-d	16-a	20-a

CHAPTER 11 - SKIN TYPES AND CONDITIONS

(Answers to Questions on Pages 48-50)

1-b	5-c	9-a	13-d	17-b
2-a	6-b	10-d	14-c	18-d
3-c	7-c	11-c	15-d	19-d
4-c	8-c	12-b	16-a	

CHAPTER 12 - HEALTH SCREENING

(Answers to Questions on Pages 51-58)

1-a	13-a	25-c	37-d	49-a
2-d	14-a	26-d	38-c	50-a
3-c	15-a	27-b	39-d	51-c
4-c	16-c	28-a	40-c	52-d
5-c	17-c	29-c	41-a	53-c
6-c	18-d	30-c	42-c	54-a
7-b	19-a	31-b	43-c	55-c
8-d	20-a	32-d	44-b	56-d
9-c	21-c	33-b	45-d	
10-c	22-d	34-a	46-b	
11-d	23-d	35-d	47-a	
12-d	24-d	36-a	48-c	

CHAPTER 13 - SKIN ANALYSIS

(Answers to Questions on Pages 59-63)

1-c	8-d	15-a	22-c	29-a
2-d	9-d	16-a	23-d	30-c
3-a	10-d	17-d	24-a	31-b
4-c	11-c	18-a	25-d	32-b
5-c	12-c	19-a	26-a	33-d
6-c	13-b	20-c	27-d	34-d
7-a	14-d	21-c	28-a	35-a

CHAPTER 14 - ANATOMY OF A FACIAL

(Answers to Questions on Pages 64-70)

1-a	11-c	21-d	31-a	41-d
2-c	12-c	22-c	32-a	42-a
3-d	13-a	23-b	33-d	43-c
4-b	14-a	24-b	34-b	44-b
5-b	15-d	25-c	35-d	45-d
6-b	16-d	26-b	36-a	46-d
7-c	17-c	27-a	37-a	47-d
8-d	18-c	28-d	38-a	48-d
9-b	19-a	29-a	39-c	
10-c	20-c	30-b	40-c	

CHAPTER 15 - MEN'S FACIALS

(Answers to Questions on Pages 71-73)

1-d	4-b	7-d	10-c	13-c
2-b	5-b	8-c	11-a	14-c
3-c	6-c	9-d	12-d	15-b

CHAPTER 16 - POSTCONSULTATION AND HOME CARE

(Answers to Questions on Pages 74-76)

1-d	5-c	9-c	13-b	17-b
2-d	6-c	10-d	14-c	18-d
3-b	7-d	11-b	15-b	19-d
4-b	8-a	12-d	16-d	

CHAPTER 17 - DISORDERS AND DISEASES

(Answers to Questions on Pages 77-83)

1-a	12-c	23-a	34-d	45-b
2-c	13-d	24-c	35-c	46-c
3-d	14-d	25-d	36-a	47-d
4-a	15-c	26-d	37-c	48-a
5-a	16-c	27-d	38-c	49-a
6-c	17-b	28-a	39-a	50-d
7-b	18-c	29-a	40-b	51-c
8-c	19-c	30-c	41-a	52-d
9-d	20-d	31-a	42-a	
10-d	21-b	32-d	43-d	
11-a	22-b	33-c	44-c	

CHAPTER 18 - PHARMACOLOGY

(Answers to Questions on Pages 84-89)

1-a	9-c	17-b	25-d	33-d
2-d	10-d	18-b	26-c	34-c
3-c	11-a	19-c	27-d	35-c
4-b	12-d	20-b	28-b	36-a
5-c	13-c	21-d	29-c	37-b
6-c	14-c	22-a	30-d	38-d
7-b	15-d	23-b	31-d	39-a
8-c	16-c	24-b	32-d	40-b

CHAPTER 19 - PRODUCT CHEMISTRY

(Answers to Questions on Pages 90-95)

1-a	10-c	19-d	28-a	37-d
2-c	11-b	20-c	29-c	38-a
3-a	12-d	21-d	30-d	39-b
4-a	13-c	22-b	31-b	40-d
5-d	14-c	23-a	32-c	41-d
6-b	15-b	24-a	33-a	42-a
7-a	16-c	25-b	34-c	43-b
8-c	17-d	26-a	35-b	44-a
9-d	18-b	27-d	36-c	

CHAPTER 20 - ADVANCED INGREDIENT TECHNOLOGY

(Answers to Questions on Pages 96-98)

1-d	4-c	7-d	10-c	13-d
2-b	5-b	8-a	11-a	14-c
3-b	6-d	9-c	12-b	15-a

CHAPTER 21- AGING SKIN: MORPHOLOGY AND TREATMENT

(Answers to Questions on Pages 99-105)

1-c	11-a	21-b	31-c	41-a
2-b	12-c	22-a	32-c	42-c
3-a	13-a	23-d	33-b	43-b
4-d	14-c	24-a	34-a	44-d
5-a	15-b	25-d	35-b	45-a
6-d	16-d	26-b	36-d	46-d
7-a	17-b	27-d	37-b	47-b
8-c	18-b	28-b	38-a	48-c
9-a	19-a	29-a	39-d	49-a
10-c	20-d	30-b	40-b	50-d

CHAPTER 22 - SENSITIVE SKIN: MORPHOLOGY AND TREATMENT

(Answers to Questions on Pages 106-112)

1-b	10-b	19-c	28-c	37-a
2-a	11-d	20-b	29-d	38-b
3-c	12-b	21-b	30-a	39-c
4-d	13-a	22-a	31-b	40-b
5-b	14-c	23-d	32-a	41-b
6-c	15-d	24-a	33-d	42-c
7-a	16-a	25-b	34-b	43-d
8-b	17-b	26-d	35-c	44-b
9-d	18-c	27-b	36-d	45-d

CHAPTER 23 - HYPERPIGMENTATION: MORPHOLOGY AND TREATMENT

(Answers to Questions on Pages 113-115)

1-c	5-b	9-d	13-c
2-d	6-c	10-b	14-d
3-b	7-a	11-c	15-a
4-d	8-c	12-a	16-c

CHAPTER 24 - ACNE: MORPHOLOGY AND TREATMENT

(Answers to Questions on Pages 116-124)

1-d	14-d	27-d	40-d	53-c
2-b	15-c	28-d	41-b	54-a
3-c	16-d	29-c	42-c	55-c
4-a	17-c	30-b	43-b	56-b
5-c	18-b	31-d	44-c	57-d
6-b	19-d	32-d	45-d	58-c
7-c	20-b	33-b	46-a	59-a
8-d	21-b	34-c	47-d	60-c
9-b	22-d	35-a	48-c	61-b
10-b	23-c	36-c	49-b	62-d
11-b	24-b	37-d	50-c	63-b
12-a	25-a	38-c	51-d	64-c
13-c	26-c	39-d	52-b	

CHAPTER 25 - ETHNIC SKIN: MORPHOLOGY AND TREATMENT

(Answers to Questions on Pages 125-129)

1-b	9-d	17-b	25-d	33-c
2-c	10-a	18-a	26-a	34-b
3-c	11-b	19-c	27-c	35-a
4-b	12-b	20-b	28-d	36-d
5-a	13-a	21-c	29-d	
6-c	14-c	22-b	30-a	
7-a	15-b	23-c	31-d	
8-b	16-a	24-a	32-b	

CHAPTER 26 - EXFOLIATION

(Answers to Questions on Pages 130-137)

1-b	13-b	25-d	37-d	49-d
2-c	14-c	26-b	38-b	50-b
3-d	15-a	27-d	39-c	51-c
4-b	16-d	28-c	40-b	52-d
5-d	17-c	29-a	41-d	53-c
6-b	18-b	30-c	42-b	54-a
7-b	19-c	31-d	43-b	55-c
8-c	20-d	32-c	44-a	56-d
9-a	21-b	33-b	45-c	
10-b	22-d	34-c	46-b	
11-d	23-c	35-d	47-d	
12-c	24-b	36-c	48-b	

CHAPTER 27 - HOLISTIC/ALTERNATIVE SKIN CARE

(Answers to Questions on Pages 138-142)

1-d	8-b	15-c	22-c	29-d
2-a	9-a	16-d	23-d	30-b
3-b	10-d	17-d	24-a	31-b
4-b	11-b	18-c	25-a	32-c
5-c	12-d	19-b	26-d	33-a
6-a	13-a	20-a	27-c	34-d
7-d	14-b	21-a	28-d	

CHAPTER 28 - ADVANCED HOME CARE

(Answers to Questions on Pages 143-147)

1-c	7-a	13-b	19-b	25-c
2-d	8-c	14-c	20-d	26-b
3-d	9-b	15-d	21-c	27-d
4-c	10-d	16-b	22-b	28-b
5-b	11-b	17-a	23-d	29-b
6-c	12-c	18-c	24-a	30-c

CHAPTER 29 - METHODS OF HAIR REMOVAL

(Answers to Questions on Pages 148-155)

1-b	13-b	25-d	37-a	49-a
2-a	14-a	26-b	38-b	50-c
3-c	15-c	27-c	39-b	51-b
4-c	16-d	28-a	40-c	52-c
5-b	17-d	29-d	41-d	53-d
6-c	18-b	30-a	42-d	54-b
7-b	19-b	31-c	43-b	55-d
8-a	20-c	32-b	44-c	56-b
9-d	21-b	33-c	45-b	57-b
10-a	22-a	34-c	46-d	58-d
11-d	23-d	35-a	47-c	
12-a	24-b	36-b	48-b	

CHAPTER 30 - WAXING PROCEDURES

(Answers to Questions on Pages 156-162)

1-a	11-c	21-c	31-b	41-a
2-c	12-a	22-d	32-b	42-c
3-b	13-b	23-c	33-a	43-b
4-a	14-b	24-a	34-b	44-c
5-d	15-c	25-d	35-b	45-a
6-c	16-a	26-c	36-a	46-c
7-b	17-b	27-c	37-b	47-b
8-b	18-a	28-d	38-a	48-c
9-a	19-b	29-c	39-d	
10-b	20-c	30-a	40-d	

CHAPTER 31 - COLOR THEORY, FACIAL FEATURES, AND SETUP

(Answers to Questions on Pages 163-170)

1-b	14-b	27-a	40-d	53-c
2-d	15-c	28-c	41-d	54-b
3-c	16-d	29-c	42-d	55-c
4-b	17-d	30-a	43-c	56-b
5-d	18-d	31-d	44-a	57-d
6-a	19-d	32-b	45-c	58-c
7-c	20-b	33-d	46-b	59-d
8-d	21-d	34-d	47-d	60-b
9-d	22-c	35-d	48-b	61-d
10-d	23-c	36-b	49-d	62-c
11-d	24-a	37-a	50-d	63-a
12-a	25-d	38-b	51-b	
13-a	26-c	39-c	52-b	

CHAPTER 32 - MAKEUP APPLICATIONS

(Answers to Questions on Pages 171-173)

1-d	6-d	11-d	16-d	21-d
2-b	7-b	12-d	17-c	22-b
3-a	8-c	13-b	18-d	
4-b	9-d	14-a	19-d	
5-a	10-a	15-b	20-b	

CHAPTER 33 - THE VALUE OF BODY SERVICES

(Answers to Questions on Pages 174-180)

1-c	12-c	23-c	34-a	45-c
2-a	13-b	24-b	35-b	46-a
3-d	14-c	25-b	36-a	47-d
4-c	15-c	26-b	37-d	48-b
5-a	16-a	27-d	38-b	49-c
6-d	17-d	28-c	39-d	50-d
7-a	18-c	29-a	40-d	51-d
8-d	19-b	30-d	41-b	52-b
9-b	20-a	31-d	42-b	
10-a	21-b	32-c	43-b	
11-a	22-d	33-d	44-b	

CHAPTER 34 - BODY TREATMENTS

(Answers to Questions on Pages 181-187)

1-c	11-c	21-c	31-c	41-d
2-d	12-b	22-d	32-c	42-a
3-c	13-a	23-b	33-c	43-c
4-c	14-b	24-a	34-b	44-b
5-a	15-c	25-d	35-d	45-b
6-a	16-b	26-d	36-b	46-c
7-d	17-c	27-b	37-a	47-b
8-b	18-b	28-b	38-b	48-d
9-d	19-c	29-a	39-d	49-a
10-a	20-a	30-d	40-c	

CHAPTER 35 - CAREER OPPORTUNITIES IN MEDICAL ESTHETICS

(Answers to Questions on Pages 188-193)

1-b	8-b	15-d	22-c	29-c
2-d	9-d	16-d	23-d	30-b
3-b	10-a	17-c	24-a	31-a
4-d	11-d	18-c	25-d	32-c
5-d	12-b	19-d	26-a	33-b
6-b	13-c	20-b	27-c	34-a
7-c	14-c	21-a	28-c	35-c

CHAPTER 36 - PLASTIC AND RECONSTRUCTIVE SURGERY

(Answers to Questions on Pages 194-202)

1-b	15-c	29-b	43-c	57-b
2-d	16-b	30-d	44-b	58-a
3-c	17-a	31-c	45-a	59-d
4-d	18-c	32-d	46-b	60-a
5-a	19-b	33-b	47-b	61-c
6-a	20-a	34-b	48-d	62-b
7-d	21-b	35-d	49-b	63-d
8-a	22-c	36-c	50-b	64-a
9-a	23-c	37-b	51-d	65-b
10-b	24-c	38-a	52-c	66-b
11-d	25-b	39-c	53-a	67-b
12-b	26-b	40-c	54-b	
13-c	27-a	41-b	55-b	
14-c	28-c	42-c	56-d	

CHAPTER 37 - PATIENT PROFILES

(Answers to Questions on Pages 203-208)

1-d	9-c	17-d	25-b	33-a
2-b	10-b	18-d	26-d	34-c
3-c	11-c	19-b	27-a	35-b
4-a	12-d	20-c	28-b	36-b
5-a	13-c	21-d	29-c	37-b
6-d	14-b	22-a	30-b	38-d
7-b	15-a	23-c	31-d	39-d
8-d	16-b	24-b	32-b	40-d

CHAPTER 38 - PRE- AND POSTOPERATIVE CARE

(Answers to Questions on Pages 209-213)

1-c	9-a	17-c	25-d
2-a	10-b	18-c	26-a
3-b	11-d	19-d	27-b
4-b	12-a	20-a	28-a
5-a	13-d	21-b	29-d
6-d	14-b	22-b	30-d
7-d	15-a	23-c	31-d
8-c	16-a	24-c	32-d

CHAPTER 39 - CAMOUFLAGE THERAPY

(Answers to Questions on Pages 214-215)

1-a	3-c	5-d	7-a	9-a
2-c	4-d	6-b	8-b	10-b